SHAMPOOING

SHAMPOOING

OR

BENEFITS RESULTING FROM

THE USE OF

THE INDIAN MEDICATED VAPOUR BATH

S. D. MAHOMED

GYAN

Published by

GYAN

Gyan Publishing House
5, Ansari Road
Daryaganj, New Delhi-110002
Phone: 011-47034999, 9811692060
E-mail: books@gyanbooks.com

Distribution Network
gyanbooks.com
India, USA, Canada, UK, Australia, France

ISBN : 978-81-212-9270-2 (PB)
First Published, 1826

2nd Impression 2023

Printed at: Gyan Press, Delhi.

SHAMPOOING
Author: S. D. MAHOMED

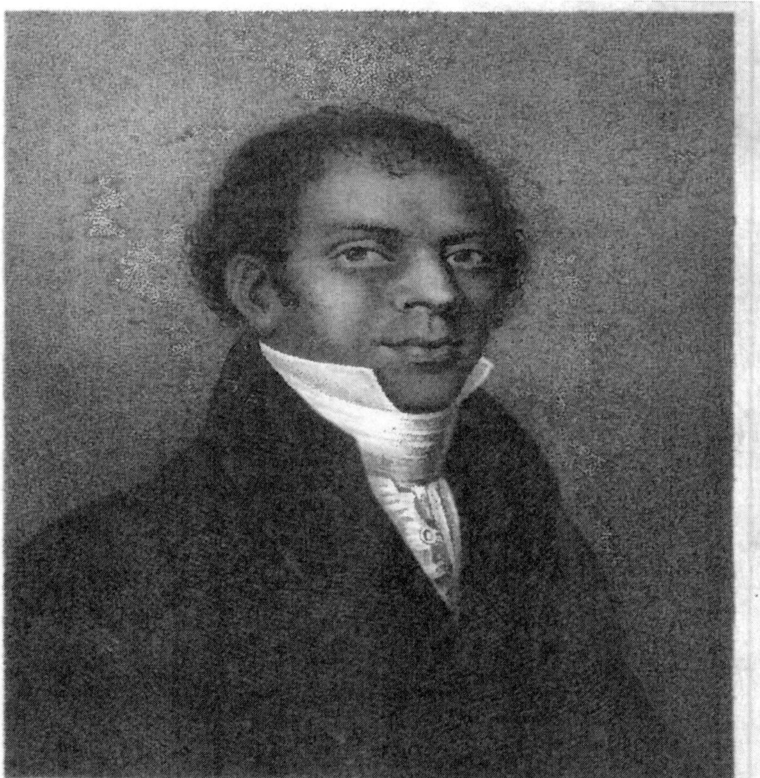

S. D. Mahomed,
Shampooing Surgeon,
BRIGHTON.

Published June 1822, by J. Cordwell at his Repository 20, Great East Street Brighton.

SHAMPOOING;

OR,

BENEFITS RESULTING FROM

THE USE OF

THE INDIAN MEDICATED VAPOUR BATH,

As introduced into this Country,

BY

S. D. MAHOMED,

(A Native of India)

CONTAINING A BRIEF BUT COMPREHENSIVE VIEW OF THE EFFECTS PRODUCED BY THE USE OF

THE WARM BATH,

IN COMPARISON WITH

STEAM OR VAPOUR BATHING.

ALSO

A detailed account of the various Cases to which this healing remedy may be applied; its general efficacy in peculiar diseases, and its success in innumerable instances, when all other remedies had been ineffectual.

TO WHICH IS SUBJOINED

AN ALPHABETICAL LIST OF NAMES

(Many of the very first consequence,)

Subscribed in testimony of the important use & general approval

OF

THE INDIAN METHOD OF SHAMPOOING.

(Second Edition.)

BRIGHTON:

PRINTED BY CREASY AND BAKER, GAZETTE-OFFICE, NORTH-STREET.

1826.

TO THE

KING'S

MOST EXCELLENT MAJESTY,

IN TESTIMONY OF

DEVOTED RESPECT,

The following sheets are

HUMBLY INSCRIBED,

BY HIS MAJESTY'S MOST DUTIFUL,

AND TRULY OBEDIENT

SUBJECT AND SERVANT,

SAKE DEEN MAHOMED.

Brighton, 1st February, 1823.

PREFACE.

I DEEM it necessary to premise, in order to be screened from criticism, that my pursuits have been widely different from those of literature, generally, through life. Little can be expected where little is promised, and my only regret is, that my endeavours will not be equal to my wishes and the expectations of my readers.

The humble Author of these sheets, is a native of India; and was born in the year 1749, at Patna, the capital of Bahar, in Hindoostan, about 290 miles N. W. of Calcutta. I was educated to the profession of, and served in the Company's Service, as a Surgeon, which capacity I afterwards relinquished, and acted in a military character, exclusively for nearly fifteen years. In the year 1780, I was appointed to a company under General, then Major Popham; and at the commencement of the year 1784, left the service and came to Europe, where I have resided ever since.

The time and attention which I devoted during the early period of my life, to the peculiar modes of Bathing, used, both medicinally and as luxuries in the Eastern part of the world, induced me to think seriously of introducing into this country that description of Bath, till then unknown, the Indian Vapour Bath combined with the Art of Shampooing; for this purpose I sedulously applied myself, when I arrived here, in trying such preliminary experiments, as from their complete success, convinced me of the correctness of the hypothesis which I had formed, that the process, which in India is used as a restorative luxury, would, with certain improvements, operate in this country also, as a most surprising and powerful remedy for many cases of disease. I felt justified in publishing to the world the discovery I had made, a discovery supported by proof the most flattering and convincing, as will be shown in the course of this work.

On my arrival in Brighton, I was not immediately enabled to promulgate the decided advantages which my method had over the common Warm-bathing; I was fortunate however, in several gratuitous cures, after every other attempt had been made and failed; cures which soon gained circulation among those who were ignorant of the virtues of my Bath, and adducing the most positive and convincing evidence of the great superiority of Shampooing over every other description of treatment, in peculiar cases.

It is not in the power of any individual to give unqualified satisfaction, or to attempt to establish a new opinion without the risk of incurring the ridicule, as well as censure, of some portion of mankind. So it was with me: in the face of indisputable evidence, I had to struggle with doubts and objections raised and circulated against my Bath, which, but for the repeated and numerous cures effected by it, would long since have shared the common fate of most innovations in science.

Fortunately, however, I have lived to see my Bath survive the vituperations of the weak and the aspersions of the credulous. Its virtues are now well known and established; it has reared itself and stands upon its own merits. We have only to refer to the cases, and a conviction of its benefits will stare us in the face.

I cannot but repeat the hope, that the following sheets may be received with that kindness and indulgence, which have ever been the distinguished characteristics of an English Public, and which will afford me a pleasing return for my humble, though grateful endeavours.

PREFACE TO THE SECOND EDITION.

Since the publication of the first edition of this work, public attention has been excited; medical men of the first professional reputation did not think it beneath their dignity, to investigate the merits of my discovery, to apply the power of reasoning to account for causes and effects; and soon were convinced of the salutary and invigorating power of the Indian Vapour Baths combined with Shampooing, if judiciously applied. Upwards of a hundred medical gentlemen have since tried the experiment on themselves; most of them were invalids, but many were merely prompted by an honorable desire to ascertain truth. By those means the Faculty in general, even on the Continent, have had their attention drawn towards my humble discovery. I feel this flattering distinction, and am in return most grateful and happy—I might add proud—when names like the following have thought proper to send patients to me.

Sir J. M. TIERNEY, M. D.	Mr. BRODIE,
Dr. HOOPER,	Mr. HEAVISIDE,
Dr. GIBNEY,	Mr. DAVIES,
Dr. THOMAS,	Mr. LAWRENCE
Dr. KING,	Mr. BOND
Dr. CLUTTERBUCK,	Mr. BARRATT,
Dr. BLAIR,	Mr. BLAKER,
Dr. GOODGE,	Mr. NEWNHAM,
Dr. ABEL	Mr. TAYLOR,
Sir H. HALFORD, M. D.	Mr. W. ATTREE, &c
Sir ASHLEY COOPER,	

With many of the most respectable members of the various branches of the healing art. I have had recommendations from two of the first Physicians at Paris; several German Physicians have visited my establishment and honoured it with their approbation. Under such auspices, it is not to be wondered at, when I assert that I could easily swell this edition with many hundreds of additional cases: but I shall only select a few which are peculiar and important. To the Public in general, and to the Faculty in particular, who with a candour worthy of their enlightened pursuits, not only appreciated the value of the invention, but at once grasped at the full capability of it, by pointing out diseases, the cure of which had not been contemplated, such as incipient pleurisy, putrid sore throat, &c. where the curative process depends principally on inhaling the warm steam ;—to all I return my most grateful thanks, and I shall, by perseverance, prove myself worthy of such signal patronage.

S. D. M.

INTRODUCTION.

ON BATHING GENERALLY.

Bathing is coeval with the remotest periods of antiquity. Homer mentions the use of private baths, which baths possessed medicinal properties, and were enriched by the most fragrant perfumes. In the eastern parts of the world, it has ever been known and esteemed, and is continued in a variety of forms, to the present period. It is not distinctly stated by any author, I believe, that the Romans directed their attention in particular to the actual cure of disease by impregnated waters, nor did they, that I can collect, imagine any virtue to result from steam immersions, or any thing beyond the simple application of water.

To the Hindoos, who are the cleanest and the finest people in the East, we are principally indebted for the Medicated Bath, in cases of disease and bodily infirmity. Many complaints to which we are subject, arise from languid circulation, and from an inactive state of the animal functions, and which in many instances resist the use of medicine, and beget consequences the most protracted and fatal; the native practitioners of India are aware of this, and Shampooing has always proved a most salutary and effective remedy with them.

B

rally speaking, less successful; this seems to be unquestionably the case in this instance, if I may draw that flattering conclusion from the exalted patronage and public confidence so generously extended to me; it is, therefore, needless to say more on this subject, since the public have, and no doubt will continue, to decide the claim to superiority, by the choice of their election.

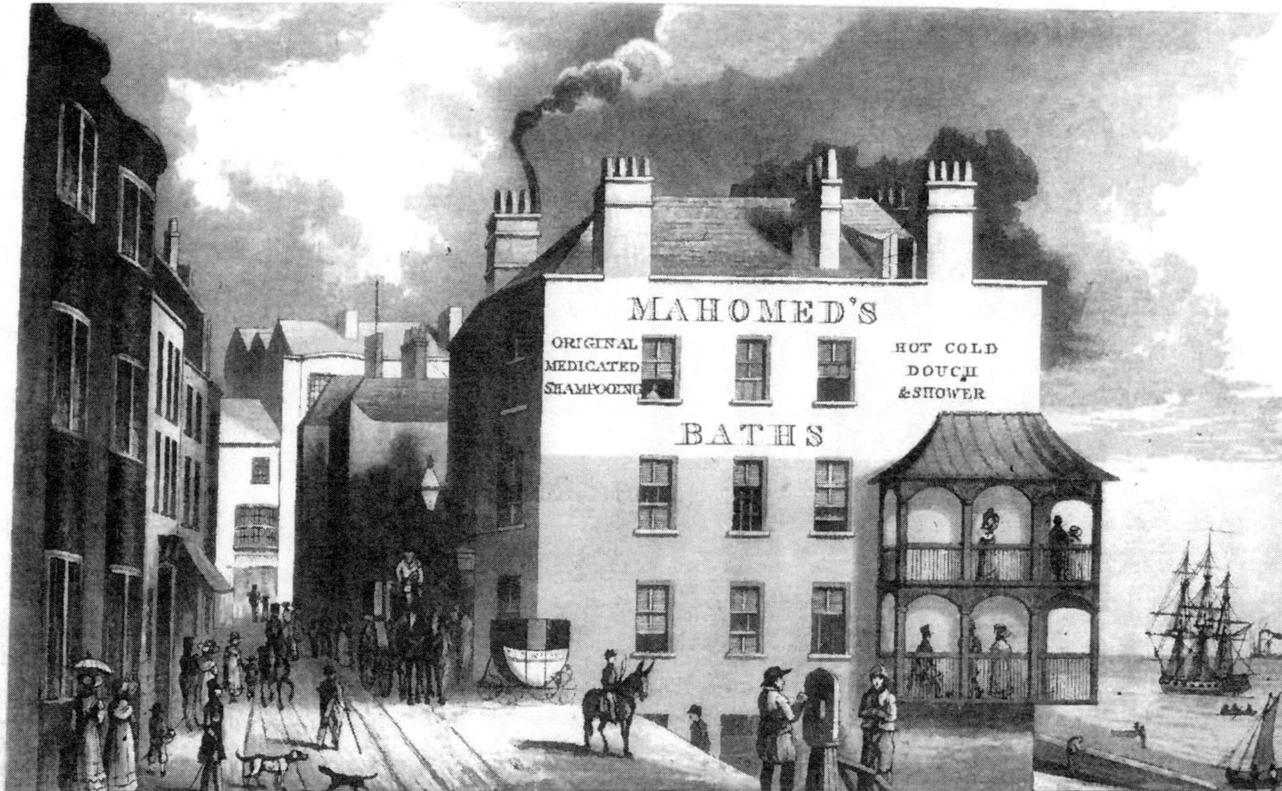
MAHOMED'S
ORIGINAL
MEDICATED
SHAMPOOING
HOT COLD
DOUCH
& SHOWER
BATHS

CHAP. I.

In the Introduction I have endeavoured briefly to enumerate a few leading particulars of the difference in effect, between Steam or Vapour Bathing, accompanied by Shampooing, and the common Warm Bath; the success which has attended my method of Shampooing, makes me desirous of laying before the public, such incontestible proofs of its general efficacy, as will confirm what I have urged in favour of the benefits resulting from its application as a concomitant on the Steam or Vapour Bathing. The cases I have arranged under separate heads, and I commence with a description of the disease, and the general mode of treatment from the best authorities, as follows:—

ASTHMA.

There are three species of Asthma;

1. *Asthma Spontaneum,* when without any manifest cause.
2. *Asthma Plethoricum,* when it arises from plethora.
3. *Asthma Exanthematicum,* originating from the repulsion of some acrid humour.

Asthma rarely appears before the age of puberty, and seems to attack men more frequently than women, particularly those of a full habit, in whom it never fails, by frequent repetition, to occasion some degree of emaciation. In some instances, it arises from an hereditary pre-disposition, and in many others it seems to depend upon a particular constitution of the lungs. Dyspepsia always prevails, and appears to be a very prominent feature in the pre-disposition. Its attacks are most frequent during the heats of summer, in the dog-days, and in general commence about midnight. On the evening preceding an attack of asthma, the spirits are often much affected, and the person experiences a sense of fulness about the stomach, with lassitude, drowsiness, and a pain in the head. On the approach of the succeeding evening, he perceives a sense of tightness and stricture across the breast, and a sense of straitness in the lungs, impeding respiration. The difficulty of breathing continuing to increase for some length of time, both inspiration and expiration are performed slowly, and with a wheezing noise; the speech becomes difficult and uneasy, a propensity to coughing succeeds, and the patient can no longer remain in a horizontal position, being as it were, threatened with immediate suffocation. These symptoms usually continue till towards the approach of morning, and then a remission commonly takes place; the breathing becomes less laborious and more full, and the person speaks and coughs with greater ease. If the cough is attended with an expectoration of mucus, he experiences much relief, and soon falls asleep. When he awakes in the morning, he still feels some degree of tightness across his breast, although his breathing is probably more free and easy, and he cannot bear the least motion, without rendering this more difficult and uneasy; neither can he continue in bed, unless his head and shoulders are raised to a considerable height. Towards the evening, he again becomes drowsy, is much troubled with flatulency in the stomach, and perceives a return of the difficulty of breathing, which continues to increase gradually, till it becomes as violent as on the night before. After some nights passed in this way, the fits at length moderate, and suffer more considerable remissions, particularly when they are attended by a copious expectoration in the mornings, and this continues, from time to time, throughout the day; and the disease going off at last, the patient enjoys his usual rest by night, without farther disturbance. The pulse is not necessarily affected in this disease, though often quickened by the difficulty of breathing. In plethoric habits, the countenance is flushed and tinged during the fit; but in others, rather pale and shrunk; in the former too, some difficulty of breathing and wheezing usually remain in the interval; in others, the recovery is more complete. On this is founded the common distinction of asthma into the humid, pituitous, or catarrhal, and the dry, spasmodic, or nervous forms. The exciting causes are various:—accumulation of blood, or viscid mucus in the lungs, noxious vapours, a cold and foggy atmosphere, or a close hot air, the repulsion of eruptions, or other metastatic diseases, flatulence, accumulated fæces, violent passion, organic diseases in the thoracic viscera, &c. Sometimes the fits return at pretty regular periods; and it is generally difficult to obviate future attacks, when it has once occurred; but it often continues to recur for many years, and seldom proves fatal, except as inducing hydrothorax, phthisis, &c.

The treatment of this disease by the faculty varies materially, and is guided in general by the nature of its appearance, and in young persons of plethoric habits, the abstraction of blood is successfully resorted to. In ambiguous cases cupping is preferable, or leeches to the chest, with blisters. Mild cathartics are also serviceably employed. Nauseating emetics have been found of great use. Squill combined with ipecacuanha, opium, fetid gum resins, smoking and chewing tobacco, strong coffee, and various other things, compounds and simples, are administered with effect at times; but much depends on the age and disposition of the patient, and more on the atmosphere as to temperature, drynesss, purity, &c. The regimen of course is a material point, and must be paid the most rigid attention to, in all stages of the disease.

Thus have I attempted a brief treatise on asthmatic complaints, and the mode of treatment resorted to by the faculty. I may now be permitted to state my remedial method, under the various and conflicting circumstances of this disease. The cases which follow will speak for me; they will prove, at least, the qualified success which has attended me in these instances, which with little difference, actuated by circumstances, were all relieved by the same *simple* means. I administered to the patient daily the Vapour Bath, prepared in some little degree different to that which I apply in other cases, and ordered him to be kept warm. "This only is the witchcraft" which I use in relieving the virulence of this disease.

In innumerable other similar cases, my efforts have been attended with the same satisfactory results, and to enter further into the mode of treatment I adopt, is, and must appear, wholly needless.

CASE 1.

Sir,—I spontaneously give testimony, under my hand, of the great service I experienced by your medicated sea-water Vapour Bath, and Shampooing. I do it the more willingly because I desire the good of others; it being a pity that such a valuable remedy should not be made public. I have been afflicted with *a bad cough and asthma,* for five years, and have been so ill for the last two months, that I could not lie down without danger of being suffocated. I lost my senses three or four times in the day, and as often at night, so that I dropped out of my chair motionless. By taking your baths a few times, I am infinitely better, and have not had a fit since.

You are welcome to make what use of this you please, for the good of others.

M. WALKER.

No. 13, New Steyne, Brighton.
Feb. 1st. 1815.

CASE II.

Dear Sir,—The great benefit I have derived from the use of the Shampooing bath, induces me to address you, not omitting my cordial thanks for the attention I received during the time I was under your care. I have been troubled with a *confirmed asthma,* for more than ten years, and have suffered greatly from the violence of the repeated attacks arising from change of situation, and from exposure to humid and thick atmospheres. During the ten years, with the exception of the last eleven months, I have never been free from the most distressing and painful fits of this disease for a month together, but, since the application of your bath, and the soothing efficacy of your method of shampooing, *I have never experienced a return* of those dreadful attacks, which rendered life a burthen—not that I mean to affirm, the malady is effectually removed, but that its virulence is considerably mitigated, and it is but justice due to you to make this candid avowal, and to acknowledge my firm conviction, that no better remedy can be applied in cases like mine, than that by which I have derived so much benefit. I was always of a weak and delicate habit, and therefore cannot say that I am perfectly in health, but, since I was first afflicted with the disease, of which you have so signally relieved me, I have never been so well and so perfectly free from pain, and all the attendant symptoms of that afflicting and terrible complaint.

I cannot too gratefully express myself for the service you have rendered me, and I trust I shall never forget your undeviating attention to me, when under your kind care at Brighton.

I am, dear Sir, yours very faithfully,

Burton Crescent, Oct. 14, 1819. T. HERON.

CASE III.

My Dear Sir,—It gives me infinite pleasure to take up my pen to return you my sincere thanks for the service you have rendered me, by the recommendation of your Vapour Bath for the amelioration of the dreadful malady under which I have so long suffered. Prior to the use of your Bath, I scarcely passed a fortnight without a fit of *asthma*, but since I first tried the Vapour, I have neither been troubled so frequently, nor so severely, as before.

If my time and occupation will allow of it, I shall pass nearly the whole of next winter in Brighton, for the purpose of trying further the virtues of your Bath and Shampooing.

I am, my dear Sir,

Yours very truly,

Oxford-street, Jan. 14, 1821. GEORGE MARTIN.

CHAP. II.

CONTRACTIONS.

My success in the treatment of this disease gives me confidence to assert, my pretensions to a knowledge of it theoretically, are not without a just foundation. In this instance, as in every other, I appeal to the testimony of the cures I have performed,—to the acknowledgment of those cures in the hand-writing of the patients themselves, (can better evidence be adduced?) to bear me out in what I advance.

There are four kinds of Contraction, viz.

1st. *Contractura ab inflammatione,* when it arises from inflammation.

2d. *Contractura à spasmo,* called also tonic spasm and cramp, when it depends upon spasm.

3d. *Contractura ab antagonistas paraliticos,* from the antagonist muscles losing their action.

4th. *Contractura ab acrimonià irritante,* which is induced by some irritating cause.

There is also another description of contraction, called *contractura articularis,* originating from a disease of the joint.

One and all of these species of disease have repeatedly come before me, and in no instance has the patient left me unbenefitted, and seldom not effectually cured. I might exceed the limits of this book, were I to venture on the different methods resorted to by the faculty, to afford relief in the various stages of this complaint: yet I challenge the most successful and effective mode practised in physic or surgery, to prove so many cases of beneficial treatment, as I can by the simple but efficacious remedy of *Shampooing*.

I will proceed at once to the evidences upon which I rest my humble claims, and which, I trust, will justify my previous assertions.

CASE I.

I, Mary Edwards, hereby declare, that in January last I was attacked by a severe cold and fever which settled in my limbs, *contracting the joint of my right knee*, so that I was wholly unable to walk, and causing the most excruciating pain:—after using Mr. *Mahomed's Baths* about fifteen times, I was greatly relieved, and am now in a rapid state of recovery.

Brighton, Sep. 12th, 1814.

CASE II.

Sir,—In compliance with your request of yesterday's date, I feel much pleasure in stating, for the benefit of whomsoever it may concern, that, in the year 1816, I was completely crippled, from *contractions in both legs*, and that from the use of your Bath for six weeks, I found myself greatly recovered. In the years 1817 and 1818, I likewise tried them again, for a shorter time—that is to say, in 1817, for a week, and 1818, a fortnight, and both times derived great benefit; insomuch, as I am now, with the exception of a little stiffness, as well as ever. Begging my best respects to Mrs. Mahomed,

I remain, dear Sir,

Your most humble servant,

EDWARD OXENFORD.

Camberwell, March 1, 1819.

CASE III.

I, Alfred Lucas, was cured of *lameness in the knee and contraction*, by a regular course of *Vapour Baths and Shampooing*, in the short space of six weeks, and have left my crutches with Mr. Mahomed.

Brighton, July 31st, 1819.

CASE IV.

Having been afflicted with a *contraction of the knee*, which was occasioned by a violent inflammation of the nerves, I was recommended to try Mr. Mahomed's *Vapour Baths and Shampooing*, which perfectly cured me in the course of three weeks.

H. GODDARD.

Upper Seymour street, Portman Square, London.

CASE V.

Sir,—My case has been considered by all who knew of it, to be a very singular one, and I hope its publication will eventually be of great use to others who may be subject to any similar affliction. For ten or twelve years I had a pain in my right arm, the strength of which gradually decreased; this I thought arose from rheumatism, until last winter, when I found myself quite disabled. I went to two eminent physicians of this town, who ordered blisters and leeches, but without effect; at length advised by a friend to try your valuable Vapour Bath (finding it not the rheumatism, as I expected) I became seriously alarmed, as the CONTRACTION assumed so formidable an appearance that I could not move my arm from my side. I must confess I was in a sad state of affliction and despondency, when I applied to you, hearing you had performed a number of wonderful cures in similar cases to mine; from the second Bath I experienced great benefit, and could move my arm comfortably, and, with a little help, raise it upon my head—*three other baths completely restored me!*

This most singular case I beg you will make public, for the advantage of the afflicted; and any further information that may be desired, will be cheerfully given to any person who may call on me for such a purpose.

I am, Sir, yours, &c.

ELIZA NEWNHAM.

49, Ship-street, Brighton.

CASE VI.

Sir,—Impressed with feelings of the sincerest gratitude for your services, it becomes a duty incumbent on me to give every publicity to the case of my sister, Maria Cordwell, who has been most miraculously cured by the application of your Shampooing or Indian Baths.

Maria Cordwell, at the age of seven years, was attacked with considerable pain and swelling in the knee, and loss of the use of her side, which none of the medical gentlemen who attended her could account for. She remained in this state *eighteen years*, receiving the advice of Drs. Garthshaw, Walshman, Pearson, Thomas, Fothergill, and Heavisides, all of whom pronounced her incurable; her knees had also become GREATLY CONTRACTED from a blister, ordered by Dr. Thomas, being on seven days, which entirely prevented her walking but with the assistance of two crutches, and then but for a very short distance,

Having fixed my residence in Brighton, and hearing daily of the numerous cures you performed, I felt anxious she should make trial of your Vapour Baths; though, from the attentions and advice she had received so many years, I must confess, I felt little hope of success,—judge then my surprise and joy in beholding her, after the short period of six weeks, walk several times up and down the room without crutches ; nay, without any assistance whatever ! She has recovered the use of her side, and her knee is so little contracted that she is enabled to put her foot to the ground and walk a considerable distance, without even the assistance of a person's arm.

This, Sir, I am proud to acknowledge to the world, is solely by the use of your Medicated Indian Vapour Baths ; and I beg you will at any time refer the afflicted to my house, where my sister will satisfy any enquiry they may please to make, and you are also at liberty to give any publicity you may think proper to this letter.

I remain, Sir,
Yours, most gratefully,
J. CORDWELL,
Drawing-master.

Repository of Arts,
19, Great East-street, Brighton.

CASE VII.

Sir,—I cannot leave this place without discharging a duty which I feel I owe to you, by thus acknowledging the great benefit which Mrs. Robinson has received under your care and direction.

Having been afflicted with *a contraction of the sciatic nerve,* she was recommended to make the experiment of Warm and Cold Sea Water Baths, but these having proved utterly ineffectual, and having been a sufferer for sixteen months, she was induced to submit her case to your opinion ; after three of your Medicated Indian Vapour Baths, Mrs. R. was enabled to lay aside her crutches and walk a considerable distance (a mile and a half) without the least fatigue or requiring any assistance. The limb is now gradually recovering its form and strength, and she remains without apprehension of any symptom of relapse. Should it be your wish to lay this simple statement before the public, I beg yon will make such use of my name as you may think proper.

I am, Sir,
Your obedient humble servant.
STEPHEN ROBINSON.

CASE VIII.

Sir,—To confess to you the extraordinary benefit I have received from the use of your Indian Medicated Vapour Baths, would be to do no more than what I have repeatedly acknowledged (viva voce) in your sitting room, to many of your patients and visitors. But, with pleasure, I can say, that I have a further object in view in thus setting forth the cure that has been performed by these Baths, accompanied by dry cupping and the usual routine of Shampooing :—it is my wish that it should be generally known, that it may give hope and confidence to the afflicted. When first I came to your Bath, I was labouring under most of those pains and infirmities that are the consequence of severe rheumatic fever and gout. Wasted in appearance—scarce able to walk—with pains arising from weakness in every joint—listless and dispirited—BOTH ARMS RENDERED USELESS BY LONG STANDING CONTRACTION—unable to help myself ;—such was my state when, trembling and with hesitation, I took my first Bath. I soon felt it a source of comfort, and suffice it to say, I that night slept without any pain, on the pillow which, the night before, it required the attention of the two nurses I was obliged to have in attendance, for a full hour, before I could be laid in a position that would give me the least hope of rest. The third Bath quite enabled me to disengage my arms from my side, to move them about in various directions, and to lift and play with the heaviest dumb-bells you presented to me—every Bath that followed gave me fresh accession of strength and freedom, and now, I am happy to say, I return to London, leaving very little to change of air and time, to restore me to a state of health, better and more complete than I have for many years enjoyed. Yes, Sir, such has been the result of your Indian Bath—the accompanying use of affriction and frequent cupping—for which I am grateful to God, and sincerely hope that this "Star of the East of our modern times, will be the means of guiding thousands from the bed of affliction, to the comforts of ease, health, and happiness. India has been the premature grave of thousands of my countrymen; it will now, I hope, make amends by sending forth that which will be the restorative to health and strength of tens of thousands.

I now dismiss the subject, with further thanks to you and Mrs. Mahomed, for kindness received, not forgetting your assistant, to whom I am under much obligation for the feeling and ability with which, under your direction, he worked the Vapour Baths.

I am, Sir, your obliged,
32, Black-lion-street, Brighton, WM. HART.
or, Royal Exchange Fire Insurance Office,
May 7, 1821.

CASE IX.

Sir,—Having heard of the cures performed by your Vapour Baths, I was induced to make trial of them. In last December I was suffering under a violent attack of St. Antony's fire in my leg and foot, attended with considerable fever, and was, in consequence, confined to my bed for near four months, so that the sinews of my leg were much CONTRACTED, accompanied with great hardness in the part principally affected, when my fever abated. I still found myself much crippled, and, for between two and three months after, I could not walk but little, and even then with the support of two sticks. In August last, I went to Brighton for three weeks, and after applying your Vapour Baths nine times, I was sufficiently restored to walk without my sticks.—I think I am in duty bound to acquaint you with this, and, if you think it may be of any use, you are at full liberty to publish this case in your forthcoming book of cures.—Sincerely wishing you success,

I am, Sir,

Your truly obedient servant,

PETER HOARE.

Carshalton, near Croydon, Surrey,
October 28, 1822.

The following names are added in further testimony of my success in the treatment of contractions :—

Antonio, Her Excellency the Countess of St., cured of contraction of the wrist.

Ashby, Miss, cured of a white swelling and a contraction of the leg.

Belton, Mrs., cured of contraction of the wrist.

Birt, Mr. George, Arundel-street, London, cured of long standing contraction of the knee.

Blomberg, the Rev. Dr., cured of contraction of the knee.

Butler, Mr. John, Cheam, cured of contraction of hip and knee.

Day, Mr. G., London, cured of a contraction of the arm.

Edwards, Miss, cured of contraction from fever.

Evans, Mr., cured of contraction of 5 years standing, occasioned by a fall from a horse.

Fowler, Miss, cured of contraction of hip and instep.

Green, Mr., cured of contraction of knee and instep.

Golding, Miss, cured of a white swelling and contraction of the knee.

Harcourt, Right Hon. Earl, cured of contraction of hip and knee.

Harriott, Mr., cured of contraction of hips and knees.

Incledon, Mr. Charles, Chedbury, Suffolk, cured of long standing contraction of the hip and knee.

Lycett, Mr., Birmingham, cured of contraction of the ancles.

Mathews, Mr., (Comedian) cured of contraction of hip and knee.

Pittock, Mr., Tunbridge Wells, cured of contraction and gout long standing.

Samuel, Mr. S., Billiter-street, cured of contraction of the knee.

Ware, Mr. S., Hampstead.

Williams, Capt., R. N., cured of contraction and debility.

CHAP. III.

PARALYSIS.

THE palsy is known by the loss or diminution of voluntary motion, affecting certain parts of the body, often accompanied with drowsiness. In some instances the disease is confined to a particular part; but it more usually happens, that one entire side of the body from the head downward is affected. The species are,

1st. *Paralysis partialis,* partial, or palsy of some particular muscle.

2d. *Paralysis hemiplegica,* palsy of one side longitudinally.

3d. *Paralysis paraplegica,* palsy of one half of the body, taken transversely, as both legs and thighs.

4th. *Paralysis venenata,* from the sedative effects of poisons. Paralysis is also symptomatic of several diseases, as worms, scrophula, syphilis, &c.

It may arise in consequence of an attack of apoplexy. It may likewise be occasioned by any thing that prevents the flow of the nervous power from the brain, into the organs of motion; hence, tumours over distension and effusion, often give rise to it. It may often be occasioned by translation of morbid matter to the head, by the suppression of the usual evacuations, and by the pressure made on the nerves by luxations, fractures, wounds, or other external injuries. The long continued application of sedatives will likewise produce palsy, as we find those, whose occupations subject them to the constant handling of white lead, and those who are much exposed to the poisonous fumes of metals, or minerals, are very apt to be attacked with it. Whatever tends to relax and enervate the system, may likewise prove an occasional cause of this disease.

Palsy usually comes on with the sudden and immediate loss of the motion and sensibility of the parts, but in a few instances it is preceded by a numbness, coldness, and paleness, and sometimes by slight convulsive twitches. When the head is much affected, the eye and mouth are drawn on one side, the memory and judgment are much impaired, and the speech is indistinct and incoherent. If the disease affects the extremities, and has been of long duration, it not only produces a loss of motion and sensibility, but likewise a considerable flaccidity and wasting away in the muscles of the parts affected.

When palsy attacks any vital part, such as the brain, heart, or lungs, it soon terminates fatally. When it arises as a consequence of apoplexy, it generally proves very difficult of cure. Paralytic affections of the lower extremities, ensuing from any injury done to the spinal marrow, by blows and other accidents, usually prove incurable. Palsy, although a dangerous disease in every instance, particularly at an advanced period of life, is sometimes removed by the occurrence of a diarrhœa or fever.

The morbid appearances to be observed on dissections in palsy, are pretty similar to those which are to be met with in apoplexy: hence collections of blood, and of serous fluids, are often found effused in the brain, but more frequently the latter, and in some instances, the substance of this organ seems to have suffered an alteration. In palsy as well as apoplexy, the collection of extravasated fluid is generally on the opposite side of the brain to that which is affected.

In the treatment of this disease, there exists great contrariety of opinion among the faculty; sometimes, where the attack is sudden, and the disease arises in the head, the patient being of a plethoric habit, copious bleeding and cupping are resorted to, and the usual means as applied in apoplexy. But where the patient is advanced in life, of a debilitated constitution and not too full of blood, an opposite mode of treatment is adopted. Many local means of increasing the circulation, and soliciting nervous energy into the affected parts, are resorted to in this complaint with various success. In all cases it is proper to keep up sufficient warmth of limb, and by what better means can this be effected than by the operation of SHAMPOOING, accompanied by the usual application of the Vapour Bath? Every physician who has written on the subject, invariably recommends the *warm* Bath, of course not knowing the nature of my process, which embraces all the soothing qualities of the common bath, added to a much greater power of emollient efficacy, and causes a quick and an active circulation locally, as it may be applied, or generally through the system. Those who have experienced its effects in instances of this disease, can never forget the relief it has invariably afforded.

I need say no more; my never failing appeal to the cases which follow, will bear me out in what I have advanced; in this disease, I may repeat with a degree of confidence, *I challenge competition from the cures which I have performed.*

CASE I.

EDWARD HENRY TULLOCH, now at Brighton, under the care of Mr. Mahomed, was, whilst at Aston Clinton, seized with a PARALYTIC STROKE, and for two years, was entirely deprived of the use of his limbs; he had been, for a long period, under the care of Mr. Ewin, of Aylesbury, and Mr. Rolles, of Tring, without being in the least benefitted by their attendance; being recommended to Brighton for the air, and there hearing of many wonderful cures performed by Mahomed, was tempted to try his remedy, and, after three times bathing only, entirely got the use of his right arm, and experienced much benefit in every respect; gained appetite, and was enabled to rest without any composing medicines; which he had not before been enabled to do.

E. H. T. still continues the Baths, and, on every fresh application, finds an increase of strength and most wonderful relief. His friends and acquaintance are astonished at the rapid change in him.

(Signed) EDWARD H. TULLOCH

Sept. 1814.

CASE II.

I, Richard Long, of Derby-place, Brighton, hereby declare, that about 14 years ago I was seized with a paralytic stroke, which deprived me of the use of my right side, and caused flying pains about my breast, head, &c. so that I was unable to walk: hearing of Mr. Mahomed's wonderful cures, I applied to him, and, by the aid of his Bath, I am in a fair way of recovery, and of being restored to perfect health.

(Signed) RICHARD LONG

Sept. 12, 1814.

CASE III.

Mr. Lee Antonee's compliments to Mr. Mahomed, and begs his acceptance of the enclosed draft, for the benefit he has experienced himself, and likewise for the waiter, at the New Steyne Hotel. Mr. Lee Antonee hopes that Mr. Mahomed may enjoy long health.

New Steyne Hotel, Nov. 10, 1814.

CASE IV.

Sir,—Having experienced much benefit from the use of your Vapour Baths, in a paralytic case, with which I have been afflicted for twelve months past, you may, if you please, refer any one to me, No. 16, Highbury Terrace, Islington, for particulars, as I shall be happy to give you the fullest testimony of my approbation.

I am, your very humble servant,

Brighton, Feb. 10, 1815. C. A. WHEELWRIGHT.

CASE V.

Mrs. Atkins, of Hinton, Yorkshire, begs to inform Mr. Mahomed of the great benefit Mr. A. has experienced from the use of his Baths. Mr: A., yesterday, without assistance, got up from his chair and walked two or three times round the room, has been out to-day, and, I have no doubt, will be enabled to walk a mile or two in a few days. Mr. and Mrs. A. are very much obliged to Mr. M. for his very kind attention.—If any reference should be, at any time, made, Mr. A. will be most happy satisfactorily to answer it.

Brighton, Feb. 17, 1816.

CASE VI.

I, Joseph Schofield, was attacked with a paralytic stroke, which completely deprived me of the use of my right knee, but, after attending the Shampooing about six times, was perfectly recovered.

No. 21, Cummin-street, Pentonville, London.

Cures, on the following highly respectable persons, have also been effected by me :—

Atkinson, Mr.
Bingham, The Hon. Mr.
Cooper, Mr.
Langharne, Admiral.
Mather, Mr., Dover.
Roddie, Captain, 38th Regiment.
Smith, Mr. Royal Artillery, Woolwich.

CHAP. IV.

RHEUMATISM.

This is a disease characterized by pyrexia, pains in the joints, increased by the action of the muscles belonging to the joint, and heat of the part. The blood, after venæsection, exhibits an inflammatory crust. Rheumatism is distinguished into *acute* and *chronic*. The acute is preceded by shivering, heat, thirst, and frequent pulse; after which the pain commences and soon fixes on the joints. The chronic rheumatism is distinguished by pain in the joints, without pyrexia, and is divided into three species; *lumbago,* affecting the loins; *ischias* or *sciatica,* affecting the hip; and *anthrodynia,* or pains in the joints. The acute rheumatism mostly terminates in one of these species.

Rheumatism may arise at all times of the year, when there are frequent vicissitudes of the weather, from heat to cold, but the spring and autumn are the seasons in which it is most prevalent; and it attacks persons of all ages; but very young people are less subject to it than adults.

Obstructed perspiration, occasioned either by wearing wet clothes, lying in damp linen, or damp rooms, or by being exposed to cool air when the body has been much heated by exercise, is the cause which usually produces rheumatism. Those who are much afflicted with this complaint, are very apt to be sensible of the approach of wet weather, by finding wandering pains about them at that period.

Acute rheumatism usually comes on with lassitude and rigours, succeeded by heat, thirst, anxiety, restlessness, and a hard pulse; soon after which, excruciating pains are felt in different parts of the body, but more particularly in the joints of the shoulder, wrist, knees, and ancles, or perhaps in the hip; and then keep shifting from one joint to another, leaving a redness and swelling in every part they have occupied, as likewise a great tenderness to the touch. Towards evening there is generally a great exacerbation, or increase of fever; and during the night, the pains become more severe, and shift from one joint to another.

Early in the course of the disease, some degree of sweating usually occurs; but is seldom so copious as either to remove the pains or to prove critical. In the beginning, the urine is without any sediment; but as the disease advances in its progress, and the fever admits of considerable remissions, a lateritious sediment is deposited; but this by no means proves critical.

Chronic rheumatism is attended with pains in the head, shoulders, knees, and other large joints, which at times are confined to one particular part, and at others shift from one joint to another, without occasioning any inflammation or fever; and in this manner the complaint continues often for a considerable time, and at length goes off.

No danger is attendant on chronic rheumatism; but a person having been once attacked with it, is ever afterwards more or less liable to returns of it; and an incurable anchylosis is sometimes formed, in consequence of very frequent relapses. Neither is the acute rheumatism frequently accompanied with danger: but in a few instances, the patient has been destroyed by general inflammation, and now and then by a metastasis to some vital part, such as the head and lungs.

Acute rheumatism, although accompanied with a considerable degree of inflammation in particular parts, has seldom been known to terminate in suppuration; but a serous or gelatinous effusion takes place.

Rheumatism seldom proving fatal, very few opportunities have offered for dissections of the disease. In the few which have occurred, the same appearances have been observed as in inflammatory fever, effusion within the cranium, and now and then affections of some of the viscera.

The faculty in the acute rheumatism, recommend the general antiphlogistic plan of treatment to be pursued, so long as the febrile and inflammatory symptoms are severe. When the patient is young, abstraction of blood, particularly when the disease attacks any important part, is necessary; but the great object after freely opening the bowels, is to procure a general and mild diaphoresis by antimonial and mercurial preparations, assisted by opium or other narcotic, which may also alleviate the pain, and occasionally by the Warm Bath, where the skin is particularly harsh and dry. Digitalis, by moderating the circulation, is sometimes usefully conjoined with these medicines. As the fever abates, and the strength appears impaired, tonics are given to promote the convalescence of the patient, and to obviate a relapse. When the disease is situated in a particular part, fomentations and other local means are employed. In the *arthrodynia*, or chronic rheumatism, the remedies of chief efficacy are stimulant diaphoretics in moderate doses regularly persevered in, assisted by various local means of promoting the circulation through the affected part. Anodynes are used both internally and locally; and the greatest attention is, or ought to be paid to the several functions of the body.

This is the mode of treatment usually adopted by the faculty: I do not dispute the efficacy of such means as are here laid down, but I have cases to prove the *inefficacy* of them in many instances: the following testimonials must speak for me again.

My success, or good fortune, or, gentle reader, call it by what name you please, has been my very close attendant on *every* case of *rheumatism* that has come before me:—I may add, I have seldom failed in affording permanent relief; and I am still led on to hope, that I may be enabled to effect even more singular services to the afflicted, than I have yet, from time and circumstances, had it in my power to perform.

CASE I.

Sir,—I have the pleasure to inform you that my son remains in good health, and happy am I to say, that I am fully persuaded his recovery, under the blessing of Providence, was owing to the use of your Vapour Bath. He had, before placing himself under your care, tried every thing the first medical practitioners could recommend, but got no relief.— It is therefore due to you, and proper for the public to know the great advantage that has resulted to him by the use of your Baths I have referred a gentleman to you this day,—his name is Hamilton. I hope your advice may prove similarly beneficial.

I am, Sir,

Your obedient servant,

WM SLARK.

16, Cockspur-street, Haymarket,
London.

CASE II.

My dear Sir,—Being now on the point of quitting this place, after a residence of six weeks, during which I have taken seven-and-thirty of your Vapour Baths, accompanied by the usual routine of Shampooing, or rubbing the limbs, for an obstinate chronic rheumatism, and general debility of system, I should esteem myself deficient, both in justice and in gratitude, were I not to leave with you a written testimony of acknowledgment of the extraordinary benefit I have experienced under your treatment, very far exceeding my most sanguine hopes.

I first waited upon you on the 28th of July last, weak, nervous, and full of anguish. I am now, by the blessing of God, and your skill, returning home stouter, more invigorated, and more free from pain than I have been for two years past. You are at full liberty to communicate the particulars of my case to any person similarly afflicted, applying to you for relief, and it will afford me real satisfaction to promote your practice, by replying to any inquiries that may be made, as to its efficacy.

I propose a journey to Brighton for a fortnight or three weeks, about the middle of November, when I shall again be a visiter at your house. In the meantime I am to be found or addressed by letter, at Walton-upon-Thames, Surrey.

Wishing you most sincerely a continuance of health and success, I take my leave, remaining always,

My dear Sir, very truly yours,

H. N. MIDDLETON.

CASE III.

To Mr. Mahomed.—I, William Edwards, Cordwainer, of No. 3, Duke's-row, Duke-street, Brighton, hereby make known, for the information of the public, that for the last three weeks I have been most grievously afflicted with the Rheumatic Gout, which deprived me of the use of my limbs, as well as of my regular rest at night. In this dreadful situation I applied to you, and, by the aid of your Medicated Baths, I have been restored to comparative health.

February 1, 1815.

CASE IV.

Brighton, July 1, 1816.

Sir,—The RHEUMATIC ATTACK in my arm having resisted every endeavour to remove it, till I had your Vapour Bath, you are at liberty to refer any person to me, in proof of its benefit. After five applications with Shampooing, and the lapse of a few days, I bathed in the sea, and continued to do so in safety; and am now about returning to London, perfectly restored.

I am, yours, &c.
CLEMENT WYATT.

Wyatt, Burkitt & Wyatt,
77, Coleman-street, London.

CASE V.

Brighton, Nov. 3, 1819.

Sir,—Considering it right that you should know the effect of your Bath, as it may be serviceable to others labouring under a similar malady, I beg to state that I brought my wife here soon after she had a RHEUMATIC FEVER, which left a violent rheumatic pain in the hip joints. After using your Bath three times, and being once cupped, she was entirely freed from the pain, and has had no return of it since.

I am, Sir, yours, &c. &c.
HENRY S. CHRISTIAN,
of London.

P. S.—I will thank you to allow the enclosed to lay upon your table for the inspection of your patients.

CASE VI.

Mrs. T. Nicoland acquaints Mr. Mahomed that she found great benefit from the use of the Vapour Bath, for the RHEUMATISM in her JOINTS.

June 14th, 1820.

CASE VII.

The following was sent to, and appeared in the *Brighton Gazette,* as an advertisement, in the month of April, 1821:

To the Editor of the Brighton Gazette.

SIR,—The following statement, in common justice, is due to the individual by whose attention the young man I am about to mention, has been restored to health, by means of the Vapour Baths and Shampooing. Moses Weymark, who lived with me, having been seized with a most violent attack of RHEUMATISM, which deprived him of the use of his legs, was advised to try the Vapour Bath; but finding its expense beyond his means, he could not for some time have recourse to it, till Mr. Mahomed generously offered him three Baths gratuitously. His state was helpless in the extreme; he was lifted from a fly; and, within an hour after the first application of the Bath and Shampooing, to my great astonishment he was enabled to walk, being, before, deprived of the least use of his legs. He continued to move about the room the whole of the day. The next morning he was sufficiently recovered to walk from the Grand Parade to the East Cliff, and after taking the Bath, walked home,—thus being quite restored in TWO DAYS, and by TWO BATHS!—That any person should have found so much relief in so short a time appears incredible. Had I not seen it, I should not have believed it; but having witnessed it, I conceive it an incumbent duty to offer it for publicity, through this medium, with the firm conviction that there is no remedy for rheumatism equal to it.

I am, Sir,
Your obedient humble Servant,
JAMES GORINGE.

Brighton, April 4, 1821.

CASE VIII.

Sir,—I cannot yet say that I am quite relieved from pain, but I have much satisfaction in attributing the whole relief I have experienced to your Vapour Bath;—and on recollection of the excruciating agony and torment my rheumatic attack brought with it, perhaps it may be an encouragement to others, under similar affliction, to recommend their doing as I have done, which I have no hesitation in saying will greatly benefit them, and, I trust, encourage your continued attention to the comforts and conveniences of your visiters.

I shall continue to recommend your Baths whenever opportunity offers; being,

Sir, your very obliged humble Servant,

WM. SHARP,

44, Weymouth-street, Feb. 23, 1822.

Mr. S. D. Mahomed, Brighton.

CASE IX.

I, John Law, of No. 3, Richmond-hill, Brighton, declare that I have been afflicted with the rheumatism in my arms and shoulders, to such a degree that I could neither dress nor undress myself for upwards of ten weeks:—being recommended to Mr. Mahomed, he applied his Indian Medicated Vapour Bath, and, after eight applications, I was restored to perfect health and strength.

February 26, 1822.

CASE X.

Brighton, Sept. 9, 1822.

Sir,—Having been afflicted with the Lumbago and Rheumatism in my back for nearly seven months, so as wholly to prevent me, for these last three months, from working at my trade,—having been, unrelieved, under several medical gen tlemen, both in London and in the country, I came to Brighton, in hope a change of air might be of service to me, when I heard of your valuable Institution, the Indian Medicated Vapour Baths :—I applied to you for advice, and I beg to say, through the kindness of God, and your humane attention to me, I am quite well and free from pain. This cure may justly be attributed to your Vapour Bathing; and as it is not in my power to recompense you for your valuable time, and the trouble I have occasioned you, I feel it in justice and in gratitude necessary to make this acknowledgment; and I give you, if you think proper, full liberty to make my case publicly known.

With the deepest sense of gratitude,

I am, Sir,

Your obedient humble Servant,

JOHN DAVENPORT.

17, Gardener-street, Brighton.

CASE XI.

London, Nov. 2, 1822.

Sir,—I feel it my duty to acquaint you, that I am quite recovered from my late severe attack of the RHEUMATIC GOUT, and have at present no appearance of relapse, which I consider almost a miracle, as you well know I was repeatedly obliged to be carried into your Bath by the assistance of two men. After taking eleven of your Indian Steam Vapour Baths I was quite restored, although I was several times given over by my friends during the operation. I must say I think the medicine (the electuary) recommended by you, and prepared under your direction by Messrs. Gregory and Bates, Chemists and Druggists, of Brighton, was of great service to me, and completely removed the chief cause of my complaint, and for-which I have to return my grateful acknowledgments. If you think proper to refer any person to me, I shall be very happy to give them any further information in my power.

I remain, Sir, yours, sincerely,

THOMAS JACKSON.

34, South Audley-street, London.

Most of the following respectable individuals have at various times received benefit in RHEUMATIC COMPLAINT by the use of my BATH and SHAMPOOING :—

Andrews, Dr.
Arthur, Mr. London.
Austin, Rev. I. Ockham, Surrey.
Barrett, Mr. Vauxhall.
Begbie, Mr. I. Hoxton.
Bentinck, Lord Charles.
Benton, Mr. G. Holborn.
Brown, Mr.
Bulbeck, Mr. John Havant.
Cleaver, Mr. S. Kennington Common.
Compton, Sir John
Cowley, Mr. Arlington Street.
Crowder, Mr. Finsbury Square.
Dallas, Mr.
Davis, Mr. Peckham.
Doyle, Sir Charles, cured of rheumatic affection and contraction of the arm.
Duval, Mr. Robert, Buckingham Street, Fitzroy Square
Eggington, Mr. Billbrook, Staffordshire.
Fairlie, Mr. Broad Street.
Fermor, Major General

Goslyn, Captain, rheumatism, five years standing, cured in three weeks.

Grey, Colonel.

Hamilton, Mr. M.P.

Herbert, Mr. R. London.

Holland, Mr. I.

Hordun, Mr. Sardon, Staffordshire.

Impey, E. Esq. Newick.

Jones, Mr. I. London.

Johnston, Mr.

Johnston, Mr. I.

Johnston, Mrs.

Kemp, T. R. Esq.

Kenny, Dr.

Lap, Mr. Cork.

Lemond, Mrs.

Liston, Mr. Comedian.

Lucas, John, Esq.

Lyons, Rev. Mr. Gloucester.

Malcolm, Sir, Pulteney.

Mathews, Mr.

Menzies, Mr. James, Edinburgh.

Morie, Mr. London.

Murray, Colonel, 18th Hussars, cured of rheumatism and contraction.

Nicholls, Mr.

Nixon, Mr.

North, Captain, R.N. Oakly, Suffolk.

Palmer, Mr. T.

Parkhouse, Mr. R. rheumatic affection and debility.

Phelan, Mr. I. London.

Philpot, Mr. Kennington.

Pitter, I. R. Bedford Street, Covent Garden.

Popham, Mr. Stamford Street.

Prater, Mr. Arlington Street, St. James.

Pugh, Mr., Brewer, Great Russell-street.
Real, Mr. Alexander, Tunbridge Wells.
Reed, Mr.
Reeves, Mr. Chas., Kennington, long standing rheumatism and contraction.
Robin, Mr. Beverston Castle, Gloucestershire.
Rodd, Capt., R. N.
Roles, Mr. Grey Coat-street, Westminster.
Rutter, Mr., Mitcham.
Schoel, Mr. John.
Shelton, Mr., Hampstead.
Simms, Mr. W. W.
Smith, General.
Sterling, G. A. Esq., Brewer-street, Russell- square.
Tayler, Mr. E. Temple, London.
Vernon, Mr., Kegworth, Leicestershire.
Whatley, Col.
Wells, Admiral Sir John.
Wigram, Charles, Esq., Fenchurch-street.
Woodthorpe, Mr., London.
Wyndham, Colonel.

CHAP. V.

SPRAINS.

A Sprain, or *subluxatio*, happens most frequently in the wrists, knees, and ankles; and is usually occasioned by a slip, or some sudden effort or violent exertion.

Sprains of the tendons and ligaments are usually productive of an immediate painful and inflammatory swelling. In severe sprains there is often not only an increased action of the arteries in the inflamed part, but there is likewise an instantaneous effusion from the rupture of some of the small vessels. In general, we may suppose the effusion to be of the serous kind, as the skin is not altered in colour for some time after the accident; but it sometimes happens that the tumid parts are either of a deep red or leaden colour from the very first, owing to blood being extravasated from the ruptured vessels.

In the treatment of sprains, two circumstances are very properly attended to by the faculty: the first, to prevent, by all possible means, the swelling from arising at any considerable magnitude; the second, to employ those remedies that are known to be powerful in removing inflammation.

To answer the first of these intentions, restringent applications, such as vinegar, ardent spirits, and the lees of red wine, are made use of. It is recommended to immerse the injured part in any of these immediately on receiving the injury; the effusion will be rendered much less than it otherwise would be, and perhaps prevented altogether. Cold water is also used soon after the accident, and is, doubtless, as a preliminary step to other applications, often attended with the best effects.

Local bleeding, leeches, and where fever is concomitant, as it sometimes is, in violent cases, opiates, together with refrigerants, and the remedies which prove useful in other inflammations producing fever, are administered. Proper rest is absolutely necessary for the limb, which never should be kept in a pendent position.

This is the usual method of treatment by the faculty; in all instances of sprain I have effected the most complete and permanent cures.

CASE I.

Brighton, Charles-street, April 25, 1820.

SIR,—It is with the greatest pleasure that I have to inform you of the benefits I have derived from the use of your Indian Shampooing Baths, after I had almost despaired of finding any restorative. I think I should be acting ungratefully and unjustly to the character of the Bath, if I did not make my case known as much as possible, for the service of others labouring under a similar complaint.

MY LAMENESS IN THE HIP arose from over exertion or a SPRAIN in riding, having travelled nearly four hundred miles in the course of a few days; I was taken ill the day after I had completed the journey (about the 21st of February, 1819,) accompanied with the most extreme pain in my right leg; in the course of a fortnight, by the constant application of Bathing Spirits, I found myself much better, when I walked from London to Chelsea, which increased my lameness very much, I was attended by a surgeon at Chelsea for some time, and then applied to Mr. Astley Cooper, who advised warm bathing and sea air. I left Chelsea for Brighton in April 1819, when I took the warm water and Vapour Bath, and continued them for four months with blisters on the hip; at the time of bathing I was electrified and cupped several times, without receiving any benefit; at this time I was not able to walk without my two crutches and a sling. I was lifted in and out of bed by two people, and attended during my stay at Brighton by four medical gentlemen:—finding no relief from them, or the bathing, I returned to town in September 1819, and continued to get much worse; my health and strength daily decreased, and the flesh on my hip, thigh, and leg, was wasting fast away; my doctors thinking me in a decline, advised my return again to Brighton for the benefit of the bathing, at which time I had two large places open on my hip, sufficient to contain sixty peas. I returned to Brighton in 1820, when hearing of your Baths, and the wonderful cures you had performed, I sent for you, and after stating my case, you told me frankly, you could make the cure in two months—I consented, and after having taken your Bath every day for nearly four weeks, I relinquished my crutches for two sticks. I now bear great weights on the leg I could not before put to the ground, my health and strength greatly improved, and my pains entirely abated, my cure may be considered as secured.

I am, Sir,
Your obedient servant,
I. H. GODWIN.

CASE II.

LORD NEWARK presents his compliments to Mr. Mahomed, and has great pleasure in stating, that his knee, which from REPEATED SPRAINS was too weak for any exertion, and almost entirely helpless, was completely restored by his Vapour Baths in three weeks, without a single drawback. He left off the *knee cap*, which he had worn for *many months*, after the second Bath.

55, King's Road, West Cliff, Brighton,
November 11, 1822.

CASE III.

Lady Louisa Cornwallis, owing to a sprain, had been unable to put her right foot to the ground for nearly two years; during that period she was attended by some of the most eminent Surgeons in London, who attributed the constant pain she suffered, to deep seated inflammation on the muscles and joints; they prescribed bleeding, blisters, vinegar poultices, and other cold applications, which were all tried without producing any amendment. Friction, warm bathing, and bandages proved equally unsuccessful.

Mr. Mahomed, upon examining her foot, felt confident the pain proceeded entirely from one of the muscles being a little twisted, and that the Vapour Bath with his method of Shampooing, would effect a complete cure.

After coming out of the Bath the third time, Lady Louisa walked across the room without support, and was at the end of ten days, able to take walking exercise for half an hour, with only slight inconvenience arising from weakness of the muscles, and is now perfectly free from the pain she suffered constantly, for more than eighteen months.

Brighton, September 17, 1822.

CASE IV.

London, Nov. 1, 1822.

Sir,—I have been requested by my sister, in compliance with your wish of adding her case to your work, now publishing, to forward you every particular of her accident and cure, feeling most happy in the opportunity thus afforded her of bearing testimony to the efficacy of your Vapour Baths, and hoping thereby to induce others, similarly afflicted, to employ the remedy which in her case has been attended with such success, the more unlooked for, as the accident occurred nearly three years previous to her applying to you. The SPRAIN IN HER KNEE arose from a very trifling cause, occasioned by her bodily health being in rather a debilitated state, and might have been less serious in its consequences, had not a very retired situation deprived her for many months of good medical advice, and it was not until after being two years on crutches that she came to London, where she remained nine months, and certainly during that time made some progress; but though hopes were firmly held out to her of a cure at last, yet not any were given of its being effected under another twelvemonth at least; during which time it was necessary to abstain as much as possible from the use of any thing that would irritate the offended nerve, and bring on a return of inflammation. Her general health in the mean time had suffered materially from confinement and want of exercise, and it was with the hope of re-establishing that, that she was first induced to think of trying your Vapour Baths. It is but justice here to acquaint you that she went to Brighton greatly prejudiced, and had fully determined not to allow the knee to be rubbed or touched in any way. In pursuance of this resolution, she took the Baths without the additional application of Shampooing, for the first week, and found her health very materially affected by them; indeed at first she was very ill, and apparently completely overcome; her knee also seemed much worse, with a return of the old symptoms of disease, heat, swelling, and pain: she however determined to persevere, and at the week's end finding her general health improving, prejudice began to give way, and she allowed her knee to be treated according to your directions, strictly following your advice in every respect: so rapid was her improvement from this time, that she could well have put her crutches aside after the eighth bath, though fear made her continue them four days longer, when she was able to walk firm and steadily without support of any kind, and step in and out of a carriage, though before obliged to be lifted as a little child. She continued the Baths after that regularly for nearly four weeks, and took in all forty, being anxious to ensure a perfect cure, from the use of which her general health derived equal benefit with the limb.

It is now five months since she left Brighton, during which time she has enjoyed an excellent state of health, though not naturally of a robust constitution, and has never experienced any inconvenience from her knee, and is now able to stand, walk, and kneel as well as ever, without either pain or stiffness. My sister particularly begs me to mention for the good of others, that in her opinion not any judgment ought to be formed of the effect of the Baths under six or eight *successive* trials in any bad case, nor can a cure be ever expected without patience and much perseverance, often in spite of discouraging appearances.

I have now only to add our united wishes for your success, and an assurance that we shall at all times feel happy in making the beneficial effects of your Vapour Baths more generally known.

I am, Sir, yours, &c.
MARIAN LE MESURIER.

The following names may be added, in further testimony of relief afforded by Shampooing, in cases of Sprains :—

Bishop, Mr. James.

Bloomfield, Right Hon. Sir B., cured of sprained knee and thigh, with lumbago.

Egremont, Right Hon. Earl of, cured of sprained wrist.

Hill, Mr., cured of violent ditto.

Tilt, Mr., 39, Paternoster Row.

CHAP. VI.

WHAT the VAPOUR BATH and SHAMPOOING, together, are enabled to effect, my readers must have had, already, sufficient proof: I do not wish to press them forward as being capable of accomplishing *every cure,* but it must be allowed on all hands, my praise of their general and conjoined efficacy, does not exceed the fair limits of truth. I have dwelt on "Asthma, Contractions, Paralysis, Rheumatisms, and Sprains:" with what success I have treated these several complaints, the letters I have received are the best testimony I can offer: I have now only to present a few cases of a general character, some of them being of a very peculiar description, and which, without comment, I lay before my readers, to bear evidence for themselves.

CASE I.

CASE OF HOARSENESS AND LOSS OF VOICE.

ANNE FOSSECK, of Gracechurch-street, London, after having taken a number of the Indian Medicated Vapour Baths, has proved their efficacy, by the restoration of her voice, which she had lost during the space of the preceding six months. This testimony she is desirous of leaving, for the benefit of others; and also, as an acknowledgment for the benefit which she has derived:

Brighton, 5th of the 8th month, 1819.

CASE II.

CASE OF VIOLENT PAIN IN THE KNEE, OCCASIONED BY A SEVERE COLD.

I, Hannah Shee, of No. 11, Mount Pleasant, Brighton, was afflicted for eleven years with a violent pain in my knee, brought on by a severe cold I caught from lying in damp sheets :—By the use of the Medicated Vapour Bath and Shampooing seven times, I was perfectly cured.

Sept. 12, 1814.

CASE III.

CASE OF LOSS OF VOICE.

Mrs. Morgan has great pleasure in acknowledging the efficacy of Mr. Mahomed's Vapour Baths, which, after a few trials, restored her voice, which she had lost for two years and three quarters.

Brighton, August 14, 1822.

CASE IV.

CASE OF SPINAL COMPLAINT.

Dear Sir,—I cannot think of leaving Brighton, without acknowledging the great benefit I have experienced by the use of your invaluable Medicated Vapour Baths, and feel truly grateful that the Almighty has blessed your system in a case where I had wholly despaired of recovery. After above four years extreme lameness from a spinal complaint, I have now the satisfaction of accompanying my friends in short walks, with the free use of my limbs ; and when I give myself the pleasure of calling on you, seeing my crutches arranged amongst numerous others on your staircase, surrendered on similar happy occasions. I assure you I have been, and still continue, a most zealous advocate in recommending invalids, and shall be solicitous to promote your interest, and contribute to the relief of my suffering fellow-creatures, by relating my own wonderful restoration.

With best respects to Mrs. Mahomed and yourself,

I remain, Dear Sir,

Your obliged Patient,

MARIAN SEDGWICK.

Brighton, May 2, 1822.

CASE V.

CASE OF DISEASED SPINE AND NERVOUS DISORDER.

Brighton, October 9, 1822.

MY DEAR SIR,—Through the divine blessing, you have been the means of so much benefit to my bodily health, that I cannot leave this place without testifying my gratitude to you upon that account.

Having from my early youth suffered severely from DISEASED SPINE, my whole constitution has received a shock which perhaps it will never altogether recover from. It is true that distressing and most painful malady was, under the judicious treatment of a very dear medical friend, nearly cured three years ago, at Clifton, that is to say, by my remaining in a horizontal posture nearly two years, the *inflammation* of the spine entirely subsided, and I was pronounced free from that disorder; yet, notwithstanding this, such a degree of weakness remained that Iwas quite unable to bear the motion of a carriage sitting up, and equally unable to bear the exercise of walking without great pain and difficulty. Some time after I left Clifton, symptoms of the disease being about to return became evident, which symptoms became more and more alarming, until I came to this place last June, at which time the curve of the dorsal vertebræ (which had never been entirely removed) became more considerable, with increasing tenderness in several of the bones. I was suffering much likewise when I came here from a very PAINFUL NERVOUS DISORDER IN THE HEAD, which made the least noise distressing to me in the extreme. Upon first using your justly celebrated Vapour Bath, the nervous irritation was greatly relieved, and my head felt more quiet and easy than it before had done for a length of time. I have now used the Bath fifty times, and can truly say that the effect has been great indeed with respect to the spine. That curve, which was so *considerable* when I came here, is *almost removed;* the tenderness, although not *entirely* removed in *all* the bones, *greatly lessened;*—I can bear the motion of a carriage *sitting up,* with comfort, which before I had not for six years been able to do;—I can now walk nearly half a mile at a time, with *more ease* than I could, when I left home, walk twenty yards. On account of the very delicate state of my lungs, I am obliged for the winter to leave the sea, which I very much regret, being well assured that continuing the Bath some time longer would quite cure the spinal disorder; however, please God I live, I hope to renew it in the spring, with increased benefit. The disorder in my head has been likewise greatly relieved, and my strength much increased, a full proof that it is not the tendency of the Vapour Bath to weaken; I can likewise bear my testimony that it does not make people grow thin, for I have been gaining flesh ever since I began to use it.

May God continue to bless you in the means you have hitherto so effectually used for the relief of your fellow-creatures; may He spare you long to your friends, and before your removal from this world, fit you for that eternal state to which we are all hastening.

I remain, my dear Sir,

Your sincere and grateful Friend,

MARY WALKER.

CASE VI.

CASE OF NERVOUS COMPLAINT, ATTENDED WITH PAINS IN THE HEAD, ALSO A CASE OF THE LOSS OF THE USE OF LIMBS.

Brighton, Nov. 6, 1821.

Mr. Mahomed.—Sir, I am very unwilling to leave your house, without acknowledging my gratitude for the wonderful cure effected on Mrs. Wartnaby by the use of your Vapour Baths and advice. She had for many years past laboured under a most distressing NERVOUS COMPLAINT, ATTENDED WITH DREADFUL PAINS IN THE HEAD, which confined her the greatest part of the year to her bed, and for which she never experienced any relief, although the advice of many medical gentlemen in London and elsewhere had been followed. About three years ago she was desired to try the effects of the sea air, and came to this place, recommended to a gentleman of the profession, who attended her for four months without the least benefit; and as I had at that time used the Vapour Baths with success in curing a long-standing head-ache, brought on, I imagine, by my constant attendance at Lloyd's Coffee-house, I much wished that their efficacy should be tried by Mrs. W ; but I was opposed by the gentleman who attended her, who seemed decidedly to object to the experiment.

Since that period she had been getting gradually worse, and at last our medical friend candidly told us that no medicine could be of service to her, and that she must keep herself wrapped in flannel, carefully avoiding all atmospheric air, and bear her miserable existence (for it was no better) with her accustomed fortitude. Seeing no end to her sufferings by her remaining in such a state, I again urged, with all the arguments I was able, the use of your Vapour Baths, and at length (though from her very weak frame not without danger) got her to your house, where she has resided for the space of two months, and now returns home with me in as good health and spirits as possible, perfectly able to bear the coldest air, and to walk for miles, if necessary.

Whilst my pen is in my hand, I take the opportunity of mentioning another most extraordinary case, recommended by me:—

A very intimate acquaintance and neighbour, who had lost the use of her limbs for the last four or five years, was induced, by my intreaties, to try your Vapour Baths, being satisfied they could do no harm—whilst at the same time her physician gave no hopes of relief—she came to Brighton, and although the Baths have only been used for a fortnight, she is now able to walk without the use of her crutches, or the assistance of any one, and doubtless will return home, in the course of a month, perfectly cured.

I remain, Sir,
Your most humble Servant,
JOSEPH WARTNABY,

Dalston, near Hackney, and Lloyd's Coffee-House.

CASE VII.

CASE OF SWELLING, AND VIOLENT PAIN IN THE LEG AND THIGH.

On the 3d of October, 1818, I was seized with a MOST VIOLENT PAIN IN MY LEG AND THIGH; a few days after which I perceived A LUMP OF HARD SUBSTANCE ON THE LATTER; ALSO A SWELLING IN THE VEINS, both of which increased every succeeding day; till, at last, I was so lame that I could not walk across the room without assistance, during the space of five weeks; nor did I ever sleep at night, the pain was so excruciating. I was ordered by a medical gentleman to apply ten leeches, which I did without receiving the smallest relief. I was then bled in the foot, without better success; after which I tried fomentations of poppies, and applied warm flannel: in short, every remedy proved ineffectual. I began to fear it would be of serious consequence, when I was most fortunately recommended to make trial of Mr. Mahomed's Vapour Baths, which I did: after the first I felt much relief; after the second I was enabled to walk up and down stairs; and, upon taking the third bath, I walked home; the *seventh* restored me to perfect health, in which state I am at present; nor have I ever felt the least pain, nor seen the smallest swelling in my veins; for all of which I certainly am indebted to Mr. Mahomed's Vapour Bath and Shampooing, and I have no hesitation in saying that I shall ever feel happy in recommending them, whenever in my power, to any one afflicted in a similar manner.

MARY DAVIS,

Servant-maid to Dr. Bankhead, Marine-parade

Brighton, Dec. 28, 1818.

CASE VIII.

CASE OF ABSCESS, ARISING FROM STRAINING THE MUSCLES OF THE THIGH.

In justice to Mr. Mahomed, I declare he has effected a perfect cure on me.—Having, from violent exercise and exertion while hunting, STRAINED THE MUSCLES AND SINEWS OF MY RIGHT LEG AND THIGH, in such a manner as not to be able to walk, A LARGE ABSCESS FORMED ON MY THIGH, and "a nervous rheumatic gout affection" (as the faculty term it) attended it, the pain of which was so great as to deprive me of rest, and I continued in this way for some months, without getting any relief, taking medicines, and being attended by the most eminent physicians and surgeons; I despaired of getting cured, and was advised to go to the sea-side, where, by accident, I heard of Mr. Mahomed. I consulted him and immediately went into his steam-bath, and found relief when I came out. I continued his bath daily—the pains left me, and I gained strength and got well; and have ever since continued so, without taking any medicine, or consulting any medical gentleman.

N.B.—It is now two years since I was so ill as I herein describe.

(Signed) SAML. HOMFRAY
Cowarth House, near Staines, Bucks,

May 1st, 1820.

CASE IX.

CASE OF VIOLENT INFLAMMATION IN THE FOOT.

Louisa Powles, daughter of Mr. Powles, of Devonshire-square, London, aged ten years, had been afflicted with a VIOLENT INFLAMMATION IN HER RIGHT FOOT, for the space of five months. She had been unable to use the foot during that period, and had suffered considerable pain and confinement. She was ordered to Brighton for the benefit of the sea air, and had been there three weeks. She bathed in the sea and warm salt-water baths; but very slight improvement, if any, was experienced. The child walked with crutches,—her right foot being suspended in a sling, unable to touch the ground, or to bear the slightest pressure upon it. At this period, Mr. Mahomed's Steam Bath was tried. After one bathing, with the process of Shampooing, the sling was thrown aside;

after two more bathings, repeated on successive days, the child walked home without her crutches; and in two or three days more, she was so far recovered as to walk a mile at a time. From that time to the present, a space of four weeks, the foot has been daily improving in strength, and the child is now on the point of returning home, able to walk nearly as well as before the inflammation appeared, with a slight limp.

During the first two days of trying the bath, the child was immersed only to the hip, under an apprehension that entire immersion might injure the general health. By Mr. Mahomed's desire, she was on the third and fourth days, wholly immersed in the Vapour. No debility whatever appeared to result from it; on the contrary, the child's general health and strength (which, however, before were good) seemed improved, and remain so to this moment. Mr. Powles thinks it right to state that he has no doubt that the child's health was in progress of recovery previously to her going to Mr. Mahomed, and that the medical treatment which she had received, and was still under, would have ended in the cure of the foot. No hopes were, however, held out to him of any other than a protracted cure; and it seems to him, therefore, that Mr. Mahomed accomplished, in a very few days, what, according to all experience and expectation, would otherwise have been the work of many months. He has, however, been very careful to state the circumstances precisely as they have occurred, for the information of others, who will, of course, draw their own conclusions from them.

J. D. POWLES.

Brighton, Sept. 12, 1819.

CASE X.

MOST INTERESTING CASE OF MERCURIAL AND COMPLICATED DISEASE.

FROM JOHN SHAW, Esq. L.L.D.

I had always been remarkably healthy and strong, but was latterly, teased with medicines, morning, noon, and night, for eighteen months; had several open sores, for the first time in my life, accompanied by high feverish pulses, generally beating upwards of 84 in the minute; during the greater part of the time, was plagued with a continued sore and ulcerated throat, violent aches and pains in my limbs, discolorations in my skin, and eruptions nearly all over me, for the last twelve or thirteen of those months, while swellings and inflammations also, occasionally appeared on my feet, ankles, hands, and fingers. For the last ten months of the same time I was confined to my house, and towards the close of that interval, ten or eleven weeks, to my bed, when my right arm was twice contracted, and right wrist nearly powerless for many days together, and two tumours fixed on my legs;—the one on the left shin burst, and the other on the outside of the right leg, above the ankle bone, was opened by incision. After Christmas, 1816, when I had been upwards of two months confined, whitlows appeared on two of my fingers, and the others were itching and inflamed round the nails, one of which had split many months before, and the roof of my mouth and inner jaws or fauces became ulcerated, on catching fresh cold.

In April, 1816, shortly after the commencement of my sufferings, my disease was said to be caused by the use of mercury, which had been administered to me in great quantities, in warm climates. In June 1816 on catching cold, I vas said to be afflicted with Saint Anthony's fire on my face, or with an ailment very like it. In the autumn of the same year, my disorder was supposed to be mingled with sea scurvy; afterwards to appear as rheumatism; subsequently as gout; and, about Christmas, 1816, as erysipelas in the mouth, and some other parts; and, more than once, it was judged by some to be syphilitic. Whatever it might have been it evidently puzzled the doctors, notwithstanding I was attended by very eminent practitioners.

Nearly exhausted by malady, in August, 1817, I was advised to discontinue medicine, to repair to the sea coast, and there to use tepid sea-water baths, and exercise in the air. I began to use the tepid sea-water bath in London, for about three weeks, in August and September, 1817, and in the middle of the latter month visited the sea-coast of Sussex; there used the tepid sea-water baths very frequently, for seven weeks, and took constant exercise in my carriage and on foot also, as far as I was able in my then very infirm state.

When I visited the sea-coast, in September, 1817, I was afflicted with œdema, or swelling of my feet and limbs; stiffness in the joints, and the remains of some of my aches and pains, especially in the first two fingers of each hand; eruptions and blotches all over my skin; scars, lumps, and corrugations on my face and forehead; my nose and lips scarred, swollen, distorted, and unpliant, as were also both my ears; sores on my palate and gums, though I had swallowed but eleven grains of sublimate, in the whole, during twenty-five days, in April, and the first fourteen days of May, preceding, and which never had provoked much ptyalism or spitting; the incision in my right leg was not healed, and large hollows remained abont the cicatrices in various parts, where there had been tumours, or ulcers; and inflammatory swellings and indurations, continued about some of those parts, and, likewise, on the first two fingers of each hand, and on and about my nose, lips, and ears; contractions also of some of my muscles and tendons, and fibrous parts distressed me; particularly the contraction of the point and lower part of the nose, which disfigured me greatly.

Having returned to London in the beginning of November, 1817, merely to shew myself to my doctors, and to consult them again, I was desired to continue the former plan of using tepid sea-water baths and exercise, on the sea-coast, and, accordingly, after a journey of three days, between London and Brighton, I visited this place, on the 15th of the same November, 1817, with all the stated ailments of the preceding September, remaining about me, and very little abated; and was not able to rise from my seat, nor to go up and down stairs, without difficulty and pain, nor was I able to walk without using a stick, and sometimes a person to lean upon: in short, I was then still dragging on a miserable existence, unfit for exertion of any kind, and unfit for the common business of life.

A gentleman, abroad, had declared to me that he speedily cured his gout by exposing only the foot and limb to steam; and one of my medical attendants had informed me that a lady was cured of obstinately returning eruptions, after several seasons' trial of the warm sea-water baths, by the use of a steam-bath, in Paris, and suggested that, perhaps, the same kind of bath might be of service to me; "but he did not know how it was used." These circumstances, and the curiosity to examine the mode of applying the vapour to the whole person, led me to Mr. Mahomed, whose painted board I recollected to have seen when in Brighton before, and, on inquiry made, I immediately resolved to try the use of the steam, and his skill.

After the first or second bathing, the œdema or swellings of my feet and limbs disappeared, and the remains of my former aches and pains ceased: at the same time, the eruptions and blotches evidently began to quit my skin, and the ragged parts of the skin became even. About the fifth bathing,

I found, to my astonishment, that the ulcers in my palate were healed, as were also those of my gums, which had been destroying the flesh for upwards of two months, without any seeming chance of being stopped by the applications prescribed. On the fifth bathing, the servant carelessly rubbed off the plaister, which had covered the sore, on my right leg, where the incision was made, and, equally to my surprise, that sore also appeared healed. The inflammatory swellings and indurations which affected my limbs and fingers, and particularly my lips and nose, quickly abated, and, before I had bathed 20 or 30 times, they were no longer perceptible. The contractions of the muscles, tendons, and fibrous parts, in and about the same number of 20 or 30 times bathing, were not to be felt, and my limbs and fingers recovered their free action, *without pain;* and my ears, lips, and nose, their proper flexibility; my joints became less stiff, and my lips and nose less distorted. The former eruptions, and such as, from time to time, have been thrown out upon my skin, during the course of bathing, have been constantly and visibly diminishing and wearing away, and the blotches have all vanished. The hollows around the cicatrices, on my limbs and other parts, have continually been filling up and becoming even with the surfaces of the other flesh. The scars, lumps, and wrinkles about my forehead, face, and other places, are smoothed. My joints have regained their suppleness; my flesh its plumpness; my skin its smoothness, clearness, and freshness: indeed, the skin has now gained a silkiness, which it has not had for years past. I have all the while been blessed with ease and lightness of spirits which I never previously experienced at any period of my life, and have been gaining strength each time of bathing: in short, after the first month of using the Steam Bath, I could walk from my lodging, on the Steyne, South Parade, up the Church-hill, and round the Church-wall, at a tolerable pace, and without slackening it, or stopping on the way, or using my stick, and prolong my walk for an hour or two without being fatigued; and I now rise from my seat without difficulty, go up and down stairs with ease, walk about uprightly, firmly, and with alertness. My nose and lips have nearly gained their original forms and appearance; and I can exert myself a good deal, apply to business with alacrity, and once more enjoy what are termed the pleasures of the world.

Wonderful also to relate,—since using the Steam Bath, I find myself so recovered, that I can read by candle light, without glasses, better than I was able to do for a long time past. On the whole, my malady has seemed to vanish under the Steam and Vapour Baths, as if by enchantment. It is my duty however to confess that (having been for several years subject to attacks of erysipelas on my left leg) my appetite failed about the third time bathing; and during the fourth day, and on the fifth, a violent attack of erysipelas, which had been preceded by the common symptoms, declared itself in the usual way, by the swelling and inflammation then appearing on my left leg, but a perseverance in the use of the Steam Bath cured the erysipelas. I endeavoured to account for the attack by damp beds on the road; bad provisions, beer, and wine, at one place; exposure to damp weather while seeking for lodgings; being heated, while last in London; on the journey, &c.; but Mr. Mahomed said, it might have been caused by the Steam Bath, because " what was in the blood must be thrown out to admit a cure."—Perhaps he was right!

I shall now answer the objections that have been made to the use of the Steam Bath. From what has been just before stated, patients should not regularly expect to be cured without an ache, a pain, some eruptions, and, perhaps, other temporary suffering or inconvenience. Happy, indeed must they be, could they fairly calculate upon escaping all such! Very many patients however may do so, but not all—consider, an emetic makes us sick at stomach; and all physic is nauseous; drawing teeth is painful, and at times dangerous; the use of the knife or lance produces pain; escharotics and caustics burn and torture us; lithotomy and amputation are horrible even to the thought; yet we submit to all these, and to be confined and teased for weeks, months, and years, in the hope *only* of a cure! Why then are patients to feel disappointment, if they be not instantly or speedily cured by the Steam Bath—especially in cases of obstinate distemper?—Or, if the improper humours be driven by the steam out of their impure blood or juices, or out of the diseased parts of the general mass, and occasion some uneasiness, or even an eruption for a few days or longer, perhaps; for surely the improper humours must be driven out, to effect the required cures: or if the steam or vapour be unpleasant to the feelings of some persons, why should they not submit to the inconvenience, as they do to the use of medicines, for the chance of a cure?

Facts and practice are better than arguments and theory—Bathing, in steam, is said to weaken and make persons lean! I have, in my own person, as well as by the evidence of other bathers, proved those assertions to be false—I bathed 64 times, in 64 following days, for nearly 30 minutes each time, and was very weak, indeed, when I began, but every day became stronger, and my flesh plumper and firmer; and it is according to reason that the warm steam bath should strengthen, and not weaken; for if the steam does occasion perspiration, it is but for a very short time, and is not that collignative, or weakening perspiration which a patient should dread, but a perspiration, or exhalation, which throws out those putrid and deadly humours and particles, from the human body, which must be expelled, in order that the disease may be gotten rid of; and the steam-bath is, certainly, the quickest, easiest, and safest method of driving those deadly humours and particles out of the human body, and sooner allows the patient, therefore, to recover strength, than the operation of any kind of physic does.—In all hot climates, hot baths have long been in common use, and instead of weakening, are known to cleanse and brace!

As to catching cold, or to feeling pains and aches, after bathing in steam, I can say that I bathed *in the depth of winter, 64 times,* exposed myself to the open air, after bathing, by using exercise, and never was before so free from cold *in winter;* and, I remarked, that I was less chilly, and bore the cold better than others who did not bathe;—my aches and pains were cured by bathing; but, if any patient should catch cold, or feel aches and pains continuing, the use of the steam bath will be the readiest cure.—I remember, Sir William Jones assured me, many years ago, that steam was a sovereign remedy for a cold in the head.

In Russia, the bathers, while warm and naked from the hot baths and stews, plunge themselves into cold water, and sometimes into rivers!!!

Folly, or interest, has circulated a report that the patient may be suffocated in the bath; and that the blood rushes to the head and the pulses are quickened therein. All these reports, I have, in my own person, proved to be false; and, if a patient could even fancy that suffocation was about to happen, the flannel, on the top of the bath, could be easily removed by the patient's own hand, even if the attendant were absent, and instantly the steam and vapour would exhale and escape, and leave the patient to breathe the free outer air of the room. Of the numbers that have used Mr. Mahomed's baths, there is not one who has been suffocated! Some have asserted that the steam will scald the patient! I have not heard an instance of it in Mr. Mahomed's baths. He can augment or decrease the quantity of steam, and increase or diminish the degrees of heat, at pleasure. There is a stop-cock just close to the feet of the patient, which, being turned, would, in an instant, check the whole of the steam from rising, and throw it off from the bath: besides, a thermometer is hung up in the bath, on which the patient may easily read and mark the degrees of heat, and, if the steam should become too hot to the feet, the patient can immediately let it escape from the bath, by throwing off the flannel from the top of the bath, as before stated.

As to the blood being turned to water by the steam, the very idea is absurd. Certainly, it must be admitted that every person and vegetable, and thing and matter in this world, is composed of the four original elements—earth, air, fire, and water; all our solid parts—as bones, flesh, &c. have water in the composition, and so has our blood, but that blood cannot be decomposed in the system, so as to be changed to water by any means. By severe and frequent bleeding, particularly, indeed, as also by various medicines, or by disease, the blood may be so impoverished or corrupted that the patient may become dropsical, or fall into other diseases; there is, therefore, great danger in frequent bleeding; for, if the famous Doctor Brown be correct, al though the scum of the blood may be restored and increased and the veins become fuller than ever sometimes after bleeding, yet the liquid with which they are then filled has not the richness of the former blood, inasmuch as the red globular particles, which are iron, are fewer, and the crassamentum or rich part of the blood, which has been taken away by the bleeding, is never restored to the system in its full purity—that happens, however, when the original blood has been drawn away from the veins; but steam cannot draw away, and, therefore, cannot leave its watery particles in the system, instead of the blood; nor can steam, like some powerful medicines, corrupt the blood by corrupting the whole human mass, and deranging the secretions and excretions, or some of them. Steam cleanses, and all that it performs is, to cause the corrupt and deadly humours and particles to be expired, or exhaled; and to aid their passage from the blood by perspiration and the transpiration of the skin; or by the expiration of the lungs, and, in the lungs, to part with its oxygen or vital air, part of which is there taken into the blood, and is necessary to refresh and purify it, as the oxygen separated by the lungs from the atmospheric air does; but the steam contains more oxygen, or vital air, and less azote, or nitrogen, or deadly and pestiferous air, than the atmosphere does, and therefore restores the health better and sooner to the patient; and, as the atmospheric air is in part composed of water, the blood, if it could be changed to water, might be so changed by the atmospheric air, as well as by steam; but that is not found to be the case, nor is it the law of nature.

All objections that I have heard against the steam-bath, appear to me to be now fully answered: but one remark I have to make respecting it, which has also been made by others, that is—that it sometimes occasions drowsiness—but it does so by composing the nerves and giving ease to the whole frame; and that, evidently, is a benefit and help to the constitution. Repose is necessary to most cures; but, if the patient in any particular case wishes to avoid it, even gentle exercise will effectually overcome the drowsiness. The bath, also, like other modes of bathing, sometimes makes the mouth dry—rinsing the mouth with cold water, or drinking a proper diluent beverage will be an easy remedy.

The vulgar adage has been quoted—" one man's meat is another man's poison,"—and it has been said—" what will cure one, will not cure all."—Steam in one way or other, by exhalation caused by the sun's heat, by the water suspended in the atmosphere, &c. &c. may be said to pervade all nature, and I look upon the use of steam as a remedy to be, therefore, an exception to those adages or sayings called general rules.—N. B.—Perhaps the steam bath would be the best method for preparing patients for common sea-bathing—for if the pores be shut up by first using the cold water, the bad humours and disease may be thereby shut up in the body, and the patient become ill in consequence; but by the pores being effectually opened by the steam, the skin is thereby prepared, so as to enable the patient to receive all the benefit of sea-bathing.

JOHN SHAW, L. L. D.
At Messrs. Heyman and Co.'s Cateaton-street,
London.

Brighton, January the 20th, 1818.

CASE XI.

CASE OF PILES.

SIR,—I had for four years been afflicted with INWARD AND OUTWARD PILES, of which, after taking your Indian Medicated Vapour Bath daily, for six weeks, and using your Indian ointment, I was perfectly cured. I think it but my duty to give you my testimony for the good of others. I had been under the care of several professional gentlemen for a considerable time, but was afforded no relief. I repeat, I am now perfectly cured.

I am, Sir,
Your most obliged servant,
JONATHAN MORGAN,
No. 3, Marine-parade, Brighton,
or Caermarthenshire, Wales.

June 17, 1822.

CASE XII.

CASE OF PAINS IN THE BACK AND LOINS.

SIR,—I had for several years past been afflicted with dreadful PAINS IN THE LOINS AND BACK, which, no doubt, proceeded from inward complaint—I conjecture either from the liver or kidnies. I applied repeatedly to members of the faculty but never found any benefit beyond a temporary relief. In the year 1821, I again experienced a return of my complaint, and suffered many days such agony that I was not able to move myself in my bed; in this situation I was induced, by the advice of several of my friends, to consult you, who advised me to lose no time in applying a Vapour Bath: accordingly I was taken to the Bath, after which I found myself a little better, and repeating them for three days, I was enabled to walk home without any assistance, but still the swelling in some parts of my body did not abate. I was then requested by you to apply a sort of fomentation, which you prepared, consisting of tobacco leaves steeped in a particular liquid, this I constantly applied for two days and nights, after which time all inflammation, swelling, pains, &c. quite left me, and I took three or four more baths, when I found myself better in health than I had been for eighteen years.

I am, Sir,
Your obedient servant,
F. CARTER.

East-street, Brighton,
Nov. 19, 1821.

CASE XIII.

CASE OF HURT THUMB.

Dear Sir,—Having resided five weeks at Brighton, I cannot possibly take leave ere I ackowledge the benefit I have derived from your Vapour Baths. Four months have elapsed since I first experienced the loss of the use of my right hand, the tendon of the thumb being violently hurt; I am now, thank God, truly happy to say I can write, and render myself every assistance.

That you and Mrs. Mahomed may long live to be a blessing to your friends and the public, is the sincere wish of,

Dear Sir,
Yours very truly,
H. NEAVE.

CASE XIV.

CASE OF INDIGESTION AND TORPID LIVER.

Miss Bright, from the Hundreds of Essex, is most happy in acknowledging the benefit she has received from using Mr. Mahomed's Vapour Bath. She had been a sufferer for several years, from INDIGESTION; and it was supposed a TORPID LIVER. After using the Bath sixteen days successively, and being cupped once in the nape of the neck, a general circulation was produced in her system; she gradually improved in health, and has every reason to hope the amendment may be permanent. In the course of nine months she used the Bath fifty times.

Brighton, July 9, 1819.

CASE XV.

I, Thomas Yeates, being afflicted with Epileptic Fits, and Weakness, for ten years, after taking ten of Mr. Mahomed's Steam and Vapour Baths, found great benefit.

CASE XVI.

CASE OF GENERAL WEAKNESS, &c.

June 26, 1822.

Sir,—I beg leave to express how much benefit I consider that I have derived from the Shampooing in your Bath. I feel my limbs, both ankles and knees, *stronger*, and I experience less fatigue in walking. It is from these circumstances that I have decided to send my bailiff down to Brighton, that he may experience the effect of your Baths. He has been very ill for a length of time, above two years, and he now suffers much pain in his arms and knees. He will be at Brighton on Tuesday, and I hope enabled to commence his course of Baths on Wednesday next. I have told him that you will regulate what is best to be done about remaining for a long or shorter period at this moment, which had better depend upon the success that attends the operation, in which I have the greatest hope, from all I have seen and myself experienced.

I am, Sir,

Yours very truly, &c.

ESSEX.

To Mr. Mahomed, Brighton.

CASE XVII.

CASE OF SEVERE COLD AND LOSS OF THE USE OF LIMBS.

(Extracted from the *Brighton Gazette* of the 30th August, 1821.)

As an additional instance of the great benefit to be derived from Mahomed's *Shampooing*, and the efficacy of such an application in similar cases to the one we are about to mention, induce us to relate the following which came under our immediate observation :—A lad, from severe cold, caught, it is presumed, by sleeping in a damp bed, that deprived him of the use of his limbs for many weeks, and which rendered him quite helpless, was recommended to try the effects of *Shampooing*—which he did, and after the *first application*, to our certain knowledge, he was enabled to walk, and did so back to the chair out of which it required the aid of two persons to assist him to the Bath! This we vouch for. We had previously heard of instances of the kind, but we were among those whose prejudices would not permit them to believe; we do now, and from the evidence we had of the invigorating and healing effects of this Eastern remedy, we shall ever be among its greatest advocates.

CASE XVIII.

CASE OF GOUTY AFFECTION AND CONTRACTION.

(Extracted from the *Brighton Gazette* of the 13th September, 1821.)

As an instance of the efficacious application of the *Vapour Bath* and *Shampooing*, as practised by Mr. Mahomed, of this town, the following case has been laid before us by an individual, whose high respectability enables us confidently to vouch for its accuracy; we give it in his own words:— "Mr. W—— was troubled for years with a gouty affection, and contraction of the right leg, so bad as to cause him to retire wholly from business; the pain felt was excruciating in the extreme, and generally prevented his natural rest at night. He was at length advised to try the effects of *Shampooing*, which he did, and in the course of ten days was comparatively restored to health; this application was continued, and after eighteen Baths he was rendered satisfactorily convalescent."—We publish this with the same motive that has induced us to allude to similar cures having been effected by this means before, and with the view o impressing the public with a just opinion of what we know to be a useful and simple remedy for many disorders to which mankind are liable.

CASE XIX.

CASE OF LONG STANDING AND CONFIRMED RHEUMATISM,

Extracted from the same respectable source (the *Brighton Gazette*) as the preceding.

To the Editor of the Brighton Gazette.

Sir,—Be pleased to give insertion to the following letter, and on my next visit to Brighton I will defray any charge you may be pleased to make.

Yours, &c.

(Signed) JOHN JOHNSON.

Mr. Mahomed,

Sir,—The great benefit which I have derived from your mode of treatment, and the apparent happiness which it has imparted to a number of my best friends, induce me to take this mode of expressing my thanks, and at the same time of promulgating the cure to your advantage, which you have so successfully effected in me. In the month of August last I was persuaded to try *Shampooing*, for a long standing, painful, and confirmed case of RHEUMATISM. I had suffered, without intermission, for six months, and had been subject to repeated attacks, during the year, for the last ten years. When I applied to you I was reduced to childish imbecility in bodily strength, helpless, and miserable, without any prospect of being relieved. Your Bath cured me in *one week*—in one week was I restored to perfect health, which I had not enjoyed for years. I was, and still feel, like a man whose constitution had been renovated—who had been touched by the magical wand of some secret power, that imparted a vigour that seemed to defy the interruption of sickness. I could scarcely walk across the room when I first applied to you;—I can now walk a mile in *ten minutes;* and, in short, possess the most perfect state of health I could wish to enjoy. To you I consider myself indebted, and to you, I repeat, I am bound to return, at least, my grateful thanks: and I feel it my incumbent duty thus publicly to express my feelings, for the benefit I have experienced by your method of *Shampooing*.

I am, Sir,

Your obedient Servant,

JOHN JOHNSON.

Haymarket, London, Nov. 1, 1821.

The following names may be added under this head, as instancing cures of various complaints, but of which I have not been furnished with authority to publish more lengthened particulars:

Adams, Mrs. benefit in case of nervous debility.

Barnes, Mr. cured of gout.

Bute, Right Hon. Marquis of, cured of case of numbness in the arm.

Carr, Mr. benefit in case of nervous debility.

Curry, Capt. cured of liver complaint.

Edwards, Miss, benefit in case of nervous debility.

Fitzgerald, Dr. Percy-street, London, cured of torpid liver.

Floyd, General, cured of gout.

Forlonger, Mr. nervous affection.

Gregory, Mr. Fordsham, Cheshire, nervous affection.

Grenville, Sir Charles, cured of sprained ankle.

Griffinhoofe, Mr. Surgeon, Hampton, Middlesex, cured of sciatica.

Hall, Mr. benefit in case of nervous debility.

Hamilton, Miss, benefit in case of nervous debility.

Harvey, Mr. cured of gout.

Hays, Mrs. cured of weakness of the knee.

Heathcote, Mr. Tottenham, nervous affection.

Hood, Sir Charles, cured of severe cold.

Innes, Mr. J. spinal case.

Johnstone, Rev. Mr. cured of gout

Jones, Miss, scorbutic attack.

Kelly, Mr. cured of gout.

Kent, Mr. C. cured of torpid liver.

Laay, Mr. benefit in case of nervous debility.

Maclean, General, cured of a case of numbness in the instep.

Mallard, Mr. Hampstead, cured of gout.

Miles, Miss, cured of inflammation of the eye.

Mills, Miss, cured of swelling in the neck.

Moleney, Mr. cured of violent pain in his bones and numbness of instep.

Oakly, Mr. cured of crick in the neck.

Oakly, Miss, cured of scorbutic attack.

Orhele, Mr John, Bury St. Edmonds, nervous affection.

Ossory, the Lord Bishop of, cured of gout in both feet and one knee.

Phillips, Mr. comedian, cured of loss of voice and violent hoarseness.

Pocklington, Mr. J. Camberwell, long standing scorbutic complaint.

Pocock, Mr. cured of piles.

Radcliff, W. cured of tightness of the chest.

Rading, Mr. benefit in case of nervous debility.

Ray, Lord, cured of severe cold.

Rediford, Mrs. cured of consumption.

Rogers, Dr. Worthing, cured of long standing sciatica.

Scott, Mr. cured of dropsy.

Smith, Mrs. cured of cancer in her breast of twenty years' standing.

Sparks, Mr. Stoke near Guildford, cured of gout.

Tusin, Mr. Limehouse, nervous affection.

Tutty, Rev. Mr. Lewes, cured of numbness in the feet.

Walkin, Miss, cured of severe cold

White, Mrs. cured of scrofula in the neck of fourteen years' standing.

Wood, Mr. cured of gout.

Woodman, John, Esq. cured of a rupture.

Wyndham, the Hon. Mr. cured of weakness of the knee and instep, from the gout.

Young, Mr. J. Brock-hill, liver complaint.

CHAP. VII.

I AM now about to add the few complimentary notices which have been taken at different times, of my humble endeavours to mitigate the sum of human suffering, and relieve the afflictions of my fellow creatures. The only gratification I can have in adding these additional pages, is that which is called forth by the unbiassed testimony afforded of the success of my practice. I hope that I may have been successful in conveying my meaning in plain and unvarnished language; and it will be an additional source of pleasure to me, if the publication of these pages may be instrumental in alleviating the condition of any one of my fellow-beings, who may be suffering under disease within the reach of my endeavours to relieve.

I have nearly concluded these sheets, which I trust will be received with all due lenity toward the imperfections which I fear they contain. Here I take leave of my readers, my patrons, and my friends, having nothing further to offer beyond the few following scraps and extracts which may not perhaps, prove unworthy of the time devoted to their perusal.

SAKE DEEN MAHOMED.

Brighton, 1st Feb. 1823.

LINES TO MR. MAHOMED,

WRITTEN BY MRS. KENT, OF WIMPOLE-STREET, LONDON.

Worn out by anguish and excess of pain,
Hope seem'd delusive and assistance vain:
Oppress'd by sorrow, languid by disease,
Depriv'd of health, all pleasure ceas'd to please;
The Bath, whose influence o'er the shatter'd frame,
Like the mild soothing of a parent came—
Bade her now hope, who felt affliction's rod,
And blest with health, now breathes her thanks to God.
To thee, Mahomed, let a grateful heart,
Its warmest thanks in gratitude impart,
By thy great skill and unremitting care,
One has been sav'd that might have perish'd here,
Who, while she feels a pulse within her veins,
Will bless thy name if memory remains.

The following Ode has appeared in *The Brighton Gazette*, *The New Times*, and several other publications.

ODE,

IN PRAISE OF STEAM,

ADDRESSED TO MR. MAHOMED,

BRIGHTON.

Begin, my Muse! the grateful theme,
And sing the wond'rous power of Steam:
See how o'er yonder foaming deep
The crowded Steam-Boats proudly sweep:
Steam's magic power oft crowds the board
Of many a high and sumptuous lord;

And in the palace too 'tis said
Steam doth its potent influence shed.
* *Bolton!* how oft we hear thy name
Resounded loud with proud acclaim:
Thy engine's pond'rous thund'ring power
O'er Britain still doth plenty shower;
While copper, bright from Cornish mines,
In current coin resplendent shines,
And urged by steam's resistless force,
Thro' England takes its wonted course.
But stay—my silly Muse, forbear,
Steam's brightest glory is *not there*;
What use are honours, plenty, wealth,
Without that best of treasures, health?
Tho' rich Golconda's glittering mine
With all its sparkling gems were thine,
Would it avail to give the joy,
If sickness were the sad alloy?
Ah no, alas!—then turn thee here,
See *Mahomed's high dome* is near!
There, there, behold the power of steam,
Of *Milton's* pen a worthy theme,
What clouds of vapour sweet pervade
That circum-ambient flannel shade,
Clouds that with health and pleasure glow
And with unequalled fragrance flow:
That vapour, like the morning dew,
Bids faded roses blush anew;
The sparkling eye and glowing cheek
Its salutary power bespeak;
Those agile limbs which freely move
O'er hill and dale, and flowery grove,
Declare, O Mahomed! the power
Of steam in thy enflannell'd bower!

---

* Mr. Bolton first employed steam-engines in coining.

Bolton ! give place—the *Indian sage*
Doth all my Muse's powers engage ;
Thou giv'st the uncertain treasure, wealth,
But *He Heaven's richest blessing, Health.*

October 8, 1822. M. W.

The following Ode appeared in The New London Magazine, I believe, in July 1822.

ODE TO MAHOMED,

THE BRIGHTON SHAMPOOING SURGEON.

Nunc opus est succis ; per quos, renovata senectus
In florem redeat, primosque recolligat annos.—Ovid.

O thou dark sage, whose vapour bath
Makes muscular as his of Gath,
Limbs erst relax'd and limber :
Whose herbs, like those of Jason's mate,
The wither'd leg of seventy-eight
Convert to stout *knee* timber :
Sprung, doubtless, from Abdallah's son,
Thy miracles thy sire's outrun,
Thy cures his deaths outnumber :
His coffin soars 'twixt heav'n and earth,
But thou, within that narrow birth,
Immortal, ne'er shalt slumber.
Go, bid that turban'd Mussulman
Give up his Mosch, his Ramadam,
And choak his well of Zemzem
Thy bath, whose magic steam can fling
On winter's cheek the rose of Spring,
To Lethe's Gulf condemns 'em.

While thus beneath thy flannel shades,
Fat dowagers and wrinkled maids
  Re-bloom in adolescence,
I marvel not that friends tell friends,
And Brighton every day extends
  Its circuses and crescents.
From either cliff, the East, the West,
The startled sea-gull quits her nest,
  The spade her haunts unearthing,
For speculation plants his hod
On every foot of freehold sod
  From Rottingdean to Worthing
Wash'd by the Esculapian stream,
Dark sage, the fair, "propell'd by steam,"
  Renew the joys of kissing
In cheeks, or lank or over-ripe,
Where time has, in relentless type,
  Placarded up "Youth Missing."
To woo thee on thy western cliff,
What pilgrims strong, in gig, in skiff,
  Fly, donkey-cart, and pillion :
While Turkish dome and minaret
In compliment to Mahomed,
  O'ertop the King's Pavilion.
Thy fame let worthless wags invade,
Let punsters under-rate thy trade,
  For me, I'd perish sooner :
Him who, thy opening scene to damn,
Derived *shampoo* from *phoo!* and *sham!*
  I dub a base lampooner.
Propell'd by steam to shake from squeak,
Mara, in Lent, shall twice a week
  Again in song be glorious,
While Kelly, laughing Time to scorn,
Once more shall chaunt "O thou wert born,"
  And Incledon "Rude Boreas."

Godwin, avaunt! thy tale thrice told,
Of endless youth and countless gold,
  Unbought "*repostum manet.*"
St. Leon's secret here we view,
Without the toil of wading through
  Three heavy tomes to gain it.
Yet oh, while thus thy waves reveal
Past virtues in the dancer's heel,
  And brace the singer's weazon:
Tell, sable wizard, tell the cause
Why *limp* poor I, from yonder vase,
  Whence others *jump* like Æson?
The cause is plain—though slips of yew
With vervain mingle, sage meets rue,
  And myrrh with wolfesbane tosses:
Still shrieks, unquell'd, the water-wraith:
That mustard-seed ingredient, faith,
  Is wanting to the process.
Dip then within thy bubbling wave,
Sage Mahomed, the votive stave
  Thy poet now rehearses:
The steam, whose virtues won't befriend
The sceptic bard, perhaps may mend
  The lameness of his verses!

LINES

ADDRESSED TO MR. MAHOMED, SHAMPOOING SURGEON, BRIGHTON.

When Nature droops and sinks beneath Decay,
When at the touch of Pain Health fades away,
Eager we fly for refuge to the art
Which bids Disease's lingering train depart,
Cheers with its beacon-light the rayless gloom,
And plucks the victim from the opening tomb,

And, blessing in its course alike and blest,
O'er the deep channels of the sorrowing breast,
Pours the ecstatic tide of Hope again,
And quells each rising fear, each struggling pain.

Long may such power, oh Mahomed ! be thine,
To the worn thousands that in sickness pine
These blessings, Heaven-directed, to impart,
And claim the homage of the grateful heart.

Brighton, 1825.

The following paragraphs are extracted principally from the BRIGHTON GAZETTE, and are merely quoted as additional evidence of the opinion entertained of the VAPOUR BATHS and SHAMPOOING, by an unprejudiced and impartial writer :—

From the BRIGHTON GAZETTE of the 2d February, 1821.

The prejudice which has existed against the Indian Medicated Vapour Baths introduced into this town by Mr. Mahomed, we are glad to acknowledge no longer exists. From the benefits derived by numerous individuals, whose general respectability places their information beyond all doubt, we are enabled to say that the most salutary effects result from this mode of bathing, and there are but few instances in which the experiment has been known to fail. The New Baths on the West Cliff, which are most spacious and elegant, we understand, were erected by a gentleman, in gratitude for the cure of a most painful and obstinate complaint, performed by Mr. Mahomed, and which only yielded to his successful mode of treatment.

From the BRIGHTON GAZETTE of the 3d August, 1821.

Mahomed, the first person who introduced the Indian Vapour Baths into this country, and which have been found of such signal utility in various diseases, is flocked to by the sound as well as the invalid, even at this season of the year: as the means of insuring or restoring health, *Shampooing* has been found equally advantageous in many cases.

From the BRIGHTON GAZETTE of the 27th September, 1821.

It is not generally known, that the celebrated comedian, Mathews, whose surgical attendants pronounced him *incurable*, and stated that he would most probably be a cripple for life, in consequence of a dislocation of the hip, occasioned by the accident of his being, some time ago, thrown out of his gig, was completely and effectually cured by Mahomed's process of shampooing; and that Phillips, the vocalist, who had lost his voice from a severe cold, by two applications of the same nature was perfectly recovered. Such are the beneficial effects of this simple, yet excellent mode of restoring and preserving health.

From the BRIGHTON GAZETTE of the 18th October, 1821.

It is remarked by Sir John Sinclair, in his Code of Health, that " there are many who keep a number of grooms to curry their horses, who would add *ten years* to their comfortable existence, if they would but employ one of them to curry themselves with a flesh brush night and morning." The currying here alluded to is, in fact, the qualified process of *shampooing*, unaccompanied with its more agreeable and medicinal properties. It is the suggestion of a man who had certainly discovered the advantages from friction being applied to the human body, but who was ignorant of the mode practised in India, where it is applied in almost all cases of disease, and where its beneficial effects are known and appreciated. It is a valuable, because it is a simple remedy, and " simples are the best restoratives," in many cases, if judiciously applied. Shampooing has performed many cures since its introduction into this country, and more particularly since its introduction into this town, for which we are indebted to Mahomed, who is alone acquainted with its peculiar preparation, and who can adduce innumerable instances of its healing virtue, and the benefits resulting from this most agreeable and renovating application.

From the BRIGHTON GAZETTE of the 6th December, 1821.

We regret to say we have not room this week to lay before our readers the case of Dr. Shaw, who was so effectually and radically cured by Mahomed. The statement is of great interest, and incontestibly proves the efficacy of the art of Shampooing in cases of extreme debility. We are also, for the same reason, unable to lay before our readers a case furnished us of a severe internal hurt, occasioned by a fall from a horse, which the never-failing process of Shampooing also effectually cured.

From the BRIGHTON GAZETTE.

The salubrity of the air of Brighton, the convenience of bathing, and the many and valuable advantages which the town possesses in other respects, both as a place of pleasure and of health, have been the means of raising it very high in the estimation of every person in the country. But nothing adds more to its importance than the excellence of its baths, and no baths are more complete, more visited, or more generally esteemed than Mahomed's, particularly his *Shampooing* Baths. This process, with little deviation, he follows after the manner of his native country. The plan is simple, merely enveloping the body in steam, arising from water, in which medicinal herbs of a most agreeable sweetness have been infused, and, rubbing the body: this application has, in many instances, performed wonders, particularly in cases of rheumatism, old sprains, and gouty affections, and in nervous and other complaints. In India, Shampooing is practised in a variety of ways.

Sir R. K. Porter, in his Travels through Georgia, Persia, &c. gives the following description of the Persian bathing process:—"The bather having undressed in an outer room, and retaining nothing about him but a piece of loose cloth round his waist, is conducted by the proper attendant into the hall of the bath; a large white sheet is then spread on the floor, on which the bather extends himself. The attendant brings from the cistern, which is warmed from the boiler below, a succession of pails full of water, which he continues to pour over the bather till he is well drenched and heated. The attendant then takes his employer's head upon his knees, and rubs in with all his might, a sort of wet paste of henna plant, into the mustachios and beard. In a few minutes this pomade dyes them a bright red. Again he has recourse to the little pail, and showers upon this quiescent patient another torrent of warm water. Then, putting on a glove made of soft hair, yet possessing some of the scrubbing-brush qualities, he first takes the limbs, and then the body, rubbing them hard for three-quarters of an hour. A third splashing from the pail prepares the operation of the pumice-stone. This he applies to the soles of the feet. The next process seizes the hair of the face, whence the henna is cleansed away, and re-placed by another paste, called rang, composed of the leaves of the indigo plant. To this succeeds the shampooing, which is done by pinching, pulling, and rubbing, with so much force and pressure, as to produce a violent glow over the whole frame. Some of the natives delight in having every joint in their bodies strained till they crack; and this part of the operation is brought to such perfection, that the very vertebræ of the back are made to ring a peal in rapid succession. This climax of skill, however, has a very strange effect to the spectator; for, in consequence of both bather and attendant being alike unclothed, the violent exertions of the one, and the natural resistance of the joints in the other, give the twain the appearance of a wrestling match. This over, the shampooed body, reduced again to its prostrate state, is rubbed all over with a preparation of soap confined in a bag, till he is one mass of lather. The soap is then washed off in warm water, when a complete ablution succeeds, by his being led to the cistern and plunged in. He passes five or six minutes, enjoying the perfectly pure element; and then emerging, has a large, dry, warm sheet thrown over him, in which he makes his escape back to the dressing-room. —The Persian ladies regard the bath as the place of their greatest amusement. They make appointments to meet there; and often pass seven or eight hours together in the carpetted saloon, telling stories, relating anecdotes, eating sweetmeats, sharing their kalions, and completing their beautiful forms into all the fancied perfections of the East: dyeing their hair and eye-brows, and curiously staining their fair bodies with a variety of fantastical devices, not unfrequently with the figures of trees, birds, and beasts,—sun, moon, and stars. This sort of pencil-work spreads over the bosom, and continues down as low as the navel, round which some radiated figure is generally painted. All this is displayed by the style of their dress, every garment of which, even to the light gauze chemise, being open from the neck to that point: a singular taste, and certainly more barbarous than becoming."

The following paragraph has appeared in most of the London and Provincial Papers.

JUVENILE FESTIVAL AT CULFORD HALL.—On Thursday the 12th ult. in commemoration of the happy recovery of the amiable Lady Louisa from a long protracted lameness (which was cured effectually by Mr. Mahomed, by the application of his *Vapour Bath and Shampooing,*) and by her desire, the children belonging to the school patronised by the Marchioness Cornwallis, ninety in number, after receiving their annual prizes, were sumptuously provided with a good dinner, consisting of plum puddings and meat pies; the young ladies at the Hall, with their accustomed benevolence and affability, waited on them, and after dinner joined them in the merry dance until tea and buns were announced to the party; after which the children resumed the trip, and kept it up until the evening was far advanced, when they retired, highly delighted with their entertainment, and grateful to their benevolent Noble benefactress. Every cottager in the village was supplied with a portion of plum pudding and meat pie that was left.

The following is extracted from the British Traveller Newspaper, of the 6th of January, 1823.

Shampooing.—The art of shampooing, now so universally known throughout England, was first introduced into this country, in the year 1784, by Sake Deen Mahomed, a native of Hindoostan, and now well known by the appellation of "The Brighton Shampooing Surgeon." The astonishing effects produced on the human frame by his peculiar method of shampooing are truly astonishing, and the wonderful cures he has performed after the skill of the faculty had failed, are the praise and admiration of all. Shampooing has now become so general that baths are established in different parts of the kingdom, by a number of individuals, and all, it would seem, upon Mahomed's principle, but we hear nothing of the cures these have as yet effected; indeed, it would appear that their method of shampooing is quite different to that of the original's, and, consequently, the result always the reverse. We understand that Mahomed is about to publish a book of the most wonderful cures he has performed within these last few years. This publication will no doubt be read with great interest.

From the Brighton Gazette.

Again we have to record an instance of the efficacy of Mahomed's infallible remedy of shampooing, in a case of extreme weakness and long standing rheumatic affection. The individual on whom this cure has been performed, is well known to us, and is truly incapable of an assertion unfounded in truth. By *fifteen* baths, he affirms, he was *radically cured* of a most painful case of rheumatism, attended by great bodily weakness.

ADDITIONAL TESTIMONIALS,

WHICH HAVE BEEN RECEIVED BY MR. MAHOMED, SINCE THE PUBLICATION OF THE FIRST EDITION OF THIS WORK.

CASE I.

CASE OF INJURED SPINE.

Thomas Hine, aged seven years, the son of Mr. David Hine, York-place, City-road, London, having met with a serious accident which affected the spine, was for eleven months quite unable to walk; several expedients were tried by the advice of different medical men, but no hope presented itself until advised to have recourse to Mr. Mahomed's Vapour Baths. In the course of a few weeks a favourable change took place, and by attending to Mr. Mahomed's directions, in a few months the boy was able to walk alone, and his parents have now the confident hope that ere long they shall see him restored to his former state. His back is grown out, but the operation of Shampooing has lessened the deformity, and there is reason to believe it may ultimately remove every defect.

CASE II.

CASE OF PARALYSIS.

Grosvenor-street, (West,) 11th Sept. 1820.

Dear Sir,—I take the opportunity of sending this letter by a friend, who is going to Brighton, to inform you that we arrived safe in town; and I know it will give you great satisfaction to hear, that Mr. Sewell ever since his return has felt himself much better, and wishes me to say "that he has most certainly derived great benefit from attending your Medicated Vapour Bath more than two months, for his great affliction under a most severe paralytic attack."

Mr. Sewell unites with me in best respects to yourself, and Mrs. Mahomed, wishing you and your children health.

I am, with esteem, Dear Sir,

Your humble servant,

ANN SEWELL.

To Mr. Mahomed.

Mr. Sewell begs you will remember him to Mr. James, for his great attention to him while attending your Vapour Bath.

King's-road, Pimlico.

CASE III.

CASE OF RHEUMATISM.

1, Cannon-place, April 21, 1823.

TO MR. MAHOMED.

SIR,—I cannot leave Brighton without expressing my thanks to you for the great benefit my daughter has experienced from the use of your Medicated Vapour Baths, the rheumatism having entirely left her, and she is able to walk four miles with perfect ease; when first she took your Baths she could with difficulty walk from room to room. Allow me once more to repeat my thanks, and believe me to remain,

Your obedient servant,

ELIZABETH PARKINSON

CASE IV.

CASE OF GOUT.

84, King's-road, Brighton, Sept. 13, 1823.

Mr. MAHOMED,—In justice to my own feelings, to you, and my sincere wish to contribute in any way towards relieving a suffering fellow being, I could not leave this, without sending you this testimony of the benefit I have received from the use of your Medicated Vapour Baths, the persevering in the use of which, has rendered my stay here most *comfortable*, and without which, I feel *assured* I should have remained as when I arrived, in a very miserable and crippled state, and unfit to have enjoyed the society of my family and friends; as you saw me, of course, I need not describe to you, the swellings and hardness in my ancle and knee joints; in short, that I could not put one leg before the other without the greatest pain and difficulty, and I began really to think I had ost the use of them, so long has an unhealthy *(I can call it by no other name,)* species of Gout been hanging about me, and I may add, though constitutionally subject to this disorder, and have suffered acute pain, it never lasted for so long a period as this last attack, and I was determined to try what a regular series of the Vapour Bath would effect. The very first I took *refreshed* me, the *second* relieved me much, and after the *third* I was enabled to walk with comparative ease and comfort. Each succeeding one had its progressive *good effect*, and now at the week's end, I can take my usual rambles, and almost forget I had the Gout *at all*. You have on your list of cases, many in every way of greater importance and consequence, quite sufficient, I should think, to prove the use and efficacy of your establishment; but as I before observed, if I can be of the slightest use to a fellow-creature, or of service *to you*, I am determined the testimony of so humble an individual as myself shall not be withheld; and with my sincere wishes for your prosperity, I remain,

Mr. Mahomed,

Your's, very much,

J. W. FERMOR, Major-General.

CASE V.

CASE OF STRAIN WITH GROSS HABIT OF BODY.

Master John Bowles, son of H. C. Bowles, Esq. of Myddelton House, Enfield, in December, 1823, from the effects of a strain with a gross habit of body to which he was subject, was obliged to be conveyed from school; his right leg was greatly swelled at the knee, and could not be put to the ground: he was attended by an eminent surgeon, who ordered fomentations and poultices to be applied: another celebrated surgeon agreed with him, that the leg should not be operated upon, but nature have its course. After six months' lingering, and walking with great difficulty by the aid of crutches, further advice was obtained from another eminent surgeon, who recommended Warm Sea Bathing, which was tried; he was brought down to Brighton in June. The Tepid Bath not being sufficiently powerful to create any great change, Mr. Mahomed recommended a trial of the Shampooing Vapour Bath, which repeated two or three times, occasioned a great discharge under the knee. By *persevering*, in a few months he was enabled, by the blessing of God, to lay aside his crutches, and before the conclusion of the year 1824, was completely restored to the use of his leg, and his bodily health being better than ever it was before. The above is a short narrative of his case, and it cannot be concluded without offering sincere and grateful thanks to Mr. Mahomed for his kindness and attention.

CASE VI.

CASE OF CHRONIC RHEUMATISM.

Sir,—You are at liberty to make use of my name in recommending your Medicated Vapour Baths, for the Chronic Rheumatism, they having cured me after suffering under that complaint for more than a year.

I am, your humble servant,

THOS. KNATCHBULL.

To Sake Deen Mahomed.

April 1st, 1824.

CASE VII.

CASE OF RHEUMATIC FEVER.

Godstone, April 16, 1824.

Sir,—The Parish Officers of Godstone with myself desire to offer to you our united very sincere thanks for your obliging attention, gratuitiously paid to Francis Fulbrook of this Parish, labouring under a severe Rheumatic attack. He has returned apparently very much mended by the treatment adopted in your valuable Baths, and is about to return to his usual work, which had been long interrupted, and it is hoped he will now be able to continue.

I am, Sir,

Your obedient servant,

C. I. HOARE,

Vicar of Godstone.

To Mr. Mahomed.

Godstone, Surrey, May 19, 1824.

SIR,—I hereby desire to return to you my sincere thanks for the unmerited favour you have bestowed on me, by the gratuitous application of your Vapour Bath, and with your permission, I desire to send a few particulars of the first attack of my disorder :—In April, 1823, I was taken with a pain in my right knee—I went to work in the morning but was obliged to give up work—I kept getting worse, and having a cold on me, I continued in pain nearly one month. I then got something better, until about the 8th day of June following—I was then obliged to take to my bed, application was then made to the Doctor, he said the rheumatic fever had seized my limbs ; I then took some medicine, and also a liquid was prepared to bathe my knees and shoulders with, but I was not able to assist in dressing myself until near the Christmas following—I then got a little better, but not likely to have the use of my arms again, (especially the left arm) but through the kindness of friends, and the application of your valuable Vapour Baths, I can now follow my daily employment with apparent ease, though I sometimes feel a small pain dart into my hips, but it is soon gone again. I sincerely desire that my case may be made known to the community at large, that all who are afflicted with the like disorder, may partake of the powerful effects of your most excellent Vapour Baths. Therefore, in gratitude for your benevolent kindness so freely shewed to me, I desire to remain,

Sir,
Your most obedient and humble servant,
FRANCIS FULBROOK.

CASE VIII.

CASE OF RHEUMATIC ATTACK AND AFFECTION OF THE LUNGS.

SIR,—Previous to my leaving Brighton, I feel it but gratitude to acknowledge the great benefit I have received from the use of your Vapour Baths, the first of which seemed completely to invigorate my whole frame, which was in a state of extreme debility, arising from a most severe rheumatic attack, as well as an affection of the lungs.

I am, Sir,
Your obedient servant,
B. TUPLING.

July 28, 1824.
To Mr. Sake Deen Mahomed.

Any reference you think proper to make to me, I shall feel much pleasure in replying to.

23, Thavies Inn, Holborn.

CASE IX.

CASE OF RHEUMATIC AFFECTION.

37, High-street, Brighton.
1st Aug. 1824.

DEAR SIR,—I beg to say you have full liberty to refer any person to me who may be similarly circumstanced to myself, or afflicted in the way I have been with a violent rheumatic affection.

Last winter after much severe suffering and confinement

to my bed for nearly two months, having tried every remedy, or professed remedy, suggested by two highly respectable practitioners, and being almost hopeless of finding relief, I was induced, at the strong solicitation of a friend, to apply to you. I did so, and having, not without, I must confess, some *reluctance* taken the first bath, (to which from my helplessness I was literally CARRIED), I found *immediate* relief; a second further relieved me, and in a few baths more, I was completely restored, thus proving, I may add, incontestibly the great benefits to be derived from the use of your *Vapour Bath* and SHAMPOOING, assisted by your excellent electuary.

I have no inducement but the public good in thus addressing you, begging you will make any use you please of this communication.

I am, dear Sir,
with many thanks for your general attention,
Your most obedient Servant,
RICHARD BISHOP.

To Mr. S. D. Mahomed,
Shampooing Surgeon.

CASE X.

CASE OF SPINAL COMPLAINT.

Miss J. Hudson begs to acquaint Mr. Mahomed, that she found great benefit from the use of his Medicated Vapour Baths, for a spinal complaint, which nearly restored her.

J. H. assures Mr. Mahomed, she will always feel much pleasure in recommending them.

Ramsgate, May 7, 1824.

CASE XI.

CASE OF SPRAINED ANCLE.

SIR,—A very severe sprained ancle, with a great distortion of the joint, for which I had been under medical advice both in London and in the country, for nearly nine months, having being cured by the blessing of God and your skill, in the *short space of Six Weeks*; I am anxious to assure you of the high estimation with which I shall ever regard your inestimable invention of the Indian Medicated Vapour Bath; and shall be most happy, whenever opportunity offers, to bear testimony to its efficacy. You are perfectly welcome to communicate the particulars of my case, and on reference to me at Walton-on-Thames, Surry, I shall have much pleasure in giving you every assistance in my power.

I am, Sir, with the warmest gratitude for my recovery to yourself, and Mrs. Mahomed,

Your obedient, humble servant,

A. M. E. HATCH.

Brighton, August 6th, 1824.

CASE XII.

CASE OF LAMENESS FROM DEBILITY.

Ship-street, Brighton,
Monday, 12th August, 1824.

DEAR SIR,—Before quitting Brighton, I beg leave to express to you my thanks, for the very great benefit I have derived from the use of the Vapour Bath, which I am happy to say, has nearly quite restored me to my former state of health. I can now walk two or three miles, without finding any other inconvenience, than a slight pain in my leg; and make no doubt I shall very shortly be entirely recovered. I shall feel pleasure in recommending your baths to my friends in town, and remain,

Dear Sir,

Your very humble Servant,

WM. HARRISON.

Mr. S. D. Mahomed,

CASE XIII.

CASE OF RHEUMATISM.

Sir,—Before I leave Brighton it is my wish, (and indeed I might add my duty) to give my testimony of the efficacy of your incomparable Vapour Bath. I came down from town to try the effect of the tepid sea bath for a rheumatic complaint chiefly felt in the feet, under which I had laboured nearly four months, my left arm from the wrist to the fingers being first attacked, and shortly afterwards rendered by swelling and pain entirely useless and obliged to be carried in a sling. On my arrival in Brighton however, I soon heard from some of my own friends such extraordinary instances of cures effected by the power of the Medicated Vapour Bath upon the human frame, that I determined upon giving that a trial instead of the sea water bath, as advised by my medical attendants in town. I could at this time scarcely walk, and even with the assistance of my servant found great difficulty and pain in hobbling a few steps before the door; after the fifth or sixth Vapour Bath I could walk without my servant's arm; and from listening to invalids in the room appropriated for their use, going into the baths or returning from them, I was astonished to hear from their own lips such miraculous accounts of cures performed upon themselves in cases so much worse than mine, that though I was gradually getting better, I felt impatient, and expected that I should more speedily recover the use of my limbs after a few *months'* confinement, when I saw before me objects perfectly restored, who had been victims of the most *obstinate* disease *for as many years.* I mention this as a caution to others not to be too sanguine; it is so natural to desire to be relieved from the only impediment to one's comfort (at least to those who are in perfect health of body) the free use of one's feet, and in a place where there are so many attractive inducements for their service. But I am convinced a great deal depends upon constitution, as well perhaps as the age of the the patient; persons of 50 must not expect that remedies can act as vigorously upon their frames, as upon those of 25; patience and perseverance I believe to be all that is required to effect a perfect restoration to health in gouty and rheumatic subjects; of this I offer undoubted authority in the person of

Sir, yours sincerely,
ROSE MOUNTAIN.

Mighell-street,
Dorset-gardens, Oct. 1, 1824.

CASE XIV.

CASE OF WEAKNESS IN THE ANCLE.

Brighton, October 2, 1824.

Mrs. Robert Page, of Kennington-road, Surry, was afflicted with a weakness in her ancle, attended with great pain, so much as to render her unable to bear her foot on the ground, and it is with great pleasure she acknowledges, that after taking Mr. Mahomed"s Vapour Bath daily thirteen times, she is enabled to walk about with the greatest ease, and without any inconvenience arising from it.

To Mrs. Mahomed, with many thanks for her kind attention.

CASE XV.

CASE OF RHEUMATISM.

Dear Mahomed,

I had intended before I had left Brighton, to have given my thanks to you personally and a hearty shake of the hand you have enabled me to put into motion, but I was prevented, and the only thing that I can now do is to bestow upon you its first efforts at penmanship.

You will be happy to hear that I bore my journey without inconvenience, though the day was damp and chilly. I could not help recalling to my mind the different state of my health at the time of my last travelling the road, the favourable change in which, under a higher power, I attribute to the trial and use of your bath.

It was about three months since that I arrived at Brighton, having for several previous months, and indeed then, suffering under a severe attack of acute rheumatism. I tried Brighton for change of air, but unfortunately, very shortly became worse, so much so, that my limbs, the use of which I had regained partially, became totally useless—with pain in every movement, and completely sleepless, I only purchased a temporary rest by the strongest opiates. In this state, about six weeks back, I proposed to my father (who is himself of the medical profession) the trial of your baths—I had heard of their success, and I wished to try them.

You may remember how I came to you helpless, hardly able to stand, dragging with pain my limbs by the help of two sticks; my general health injured, and indeed, almost worn out. I tried one Vapour Bath, and that night, for the first time for many months, enjoyed a refreshing sleep, and I awoke with agreeable ease and freedom in my limbs, and from that time to the present, I have never had occasion to use my accustomed opiates. Were it only that your bath produced so great a blessing as sleep, it would be of itself a sufficient recommendation to all invalids to make use of it to regain so desirable an object. But it did more; in a few more baths my spirits recovered; my movements became easier—I soon walked, and I may now, after nine baths, confidently hope, as I gather fresh strength every day, that though late in the season, the relief that you afforded me will be permanent, and that I shall be completely restored to my former health and strength.

So assured am I of the efficacy of your Vapour Bath in the rheumatism, even in the worst form, by my own case, that

I shall feel happy if any representations of mine in this letter, if you think proper to make use of it, will induce any afflicted with it, to use so speedy, and simple, and, as I have found, so effectual a remedy to their sufferings.

I am, dear Mahomed,

Yours thankfully,

W. BODHAM WRIGHT.

3, Grenville-street, Brunswick-square.

P. S.—Please to thank your son for me, for his kind attention when I was helpless.

CASE XVI.

TO MR. MAHOMED.

CASE OF COMPLICATED DISEASE.

Dear Sir,—Having received the great benefit which I have from your able treatment of me, aided by the use of your Shampooing Baths, I feel it but my duty thus to state my case, in order that you may, if you please, make use of it in any future edition of your work.

Before I applied to you I had been suffering many years under a complication of disorders, and none of them of the least virulent kind. I was reduced to a skeleton, and, in fact, was one mass of disease; my imbecilities could only be equalled by a suspension of all my bodily faculties; I was wretched and miserable, an incumbrance to myself and to my friends. After the use of your Baths for a few times, and experiencing your kind attention for two or three days only, I began to be relieved of pain; the inflammation in my joints began to subside, and, in short, I began gradually to mend!! Having had about 30 Baths in the course of six weeks, aided by the use of your Indian electuary, I was entirely cured, and am as well and as strong as ever I was in my life.

I repeat, this letter and acknowledgment to be but a duty I owe you and the public, if you think proper to give it publicity.

I am, dear Sir,
Your's truly,
GEORGE DROWLEY.

Lewes, Oct. 29, 1824.

CASE XVII.

CASE OF LAMENESS FROM DEBILITY.

12, Broad-street.

Dear Sir.—Had you not requested from me a written acknowledgment of the utility of your Vapour Baths, my own feelings would never have allowed me to quit this neighbourhood without leaving one; and the more especially as every additional testimony to the efficacy of your plan may lead to its more general adoption, and thereby further your own interests, as well as the health of other individuals. It may be satisfactory to others, and gratifying to you, to state that previous to my coming to Brighton, I had been confined for nearly three months with a total lameness in the left foot, which was considered by several medical gentlemen of respectability to proceed from either a sprain, or constitutional debility. On my arrival here I took the warm baths for three weeks, and was not sensible of the least amendment; I then was recommended by our own medical man to try your Vapour and Shampooing Baths: I visited you, when you gave it as your opinion that the nerve of the foot was chilled. After the first bath I took I could stand with a stick, though I had not put my foot to the ground for three months; after the second I walked for half an hour; I pursued your plan for three weeks only, and I am most happy and grateful to say that I am now perfectly restored, and am able to walk a mile or two in the day, without any inconvenience. With best wishes for the health and prosperity of yourself and family, I remain, Sir,

Yours, most respectfully and obliged,

JUDITH HAGUE.

My place of residence is Tottenham Brook Place, Middlesex.

CASE XVIII.

CASE OF SPRAIN AND INFLAMMATION OF THE KNEE.

Mr. Winstgatt, Merton Cottage, Surrey, cured of violent inflammation of the knee and tightness of the tendons, occasioned by a fall, and of more than a year's standing, after applying one general and ten local Baths, at Mr. Mahomed's.

Brighton, Nov. 19, 1824.

CASE XIX.

CASE OF STRAIN WITH ABSCESS.

Brighton, December 22, 1824.

Dear Sir,—According to your desire I leave you the particulars in writing of my case.

It is now nearly six years since I first felt symptoms of a strain in the left thigh. Surgical advice was applied to, but little was thought of it, until about six months after an abscess was found to have formed between the muscles.

The course which had been recommended, not tending to check it, it had greatly extended on all sides. It was opened, and in time it healed, but was far from cured. Not to trouble you with an account of the relapses, I shall merely say, that under the treatment which was pursued, it continued for a long time growing worse, when getting into other hands, by very skilful treatment the abscess was removed: but the limb had been so much injured, that I was left without hope of ever regaining the use of it. Reduced to a state of extreme weakness, without power to bend the knee or raise the foot from the ground, the muscles of the thigh in some parts destroyed, and in others, adhering one to another and to the bone, and unable with crutches to walk more than a few yards without great fatigue. I was advised by Mr. Brodie to try your Medicated Vapour Baths; I have done so, and the result is, that I have thrown off the crutches, and am now able to walk a mile or two with ease and safety. The muscles, the knee, and all parts of the limb, have nearly regained their proper action, and I have every prospect of still further improvement.

With pleasure I take this opportunity of again expressing to you my gratitude, for the benefit I have derived from your invaluable Baths.

I am, Sir,
Your's truly,
ARTHUR SAVAGE.

To Mr. Mahomed, Brighton.

CASE XX.

CASE OF RHEUMATISM.

TO SAKE DEEN MAHOMED.

Sir,—Being under the necessity of leaving Brighton early to-morrow morning, after a residence here of about twenty days, during which time I have taken seven of your Vapour Baths, with the usual method of Shampooing, for a severe attack of rheumatism, I should think myself wanting in common justice to you, were I not to leave behind me a written testimony of the very great benefit I have experienced under your treatment.

When I first saw you, I was suffering so dreadfully from pain in the joints, that I could scarcely walk, even with the assistance of a stick : and I am now, by the blessing of God, and your skill, almost entirely free from all pain, and can walk as well as ever I could. You are at liberty to make known the particulars of my case, and I shall have much pleasure in replying to any inquiries that may be made as to the efficacy of your system. I am to be found or addressed by letter, at Walton-grove, Walton-upon-Thames, Surry—or at 39, Welbeck-street, Cavendish-square, London.

I remain, Sir.
Your obedient servant,
GEORGE BLAIR.

CASE XXI.

CASE OF RHEUMATISM.

German-place, Friday.

My Dear Sir,—Be so good as to send by the bearer, as much of your valuable medicated oil as you can spare, that you may finish that cure, you have so admirably begun. The bearer will pay the expence with pleasure.

I am obliged to return to town to-morrow—my address is No. 51, Pall Mall, where I have resided these 40 years—and from whence I will take the liberty of corresponding with you, upon the subject of my miserable rheumatic complaint, in which your good advice has already been of so much use to me. Believe me ever,

My dear Sir,
Your obedient and obliged servant,
GEORGE NICOL.

CASE XXII.

CASE OF CONTRACTION OF THE KNEE.

Mr. R. Dean was by Mahomed's Vapour Baths, enabled to lay aside his crutches, after having been compelled to use them for above TWO YEARS, in the month of February, 1825.

CASE XXIII.

CASE OF CONTRACTION AND INFLAMMATION OF THE KNEE.

I, William Gilfin, leave this as a testimony of the great benefit I have received from your valuable Vapour Bath; when I came to Brighton, I was obliged to have a Fly to come and go from the bath, but after a short stay of one month, I could walk to the bath or any other part of Brighton, with one under-hand stick; my case was a bad knee, contracted with an inflammation, of which I had been lame six months. This is perfectly at your service to publish, if you think it worthy of a place in your book of cases of cures.

WILLIAM GILFIN.

Guestling, near Hastings, Sussex.
March 7, 1825.
To Mr. S. D. Mahomed, Brighton.

CASE XXIV.

CASE OF TIC DOULOUREUX AND RHEUMATISM.

Paris, 6 Avril, 1825.

Je commence, Monsieur, par vous remercier de la petite fiole de votre huile qui accompagnoit votre lettre du 15 Mars, et vous prier de vouloir bien, aussitot que vous aurez reçu la nouvelle cargaison que vous attendez des Indes, m'envoyer, ainsi que vous me le promettiez, une petite provision de votre huile, c'est à dire de la plus forte des deux. Comme vous n'avez jamais voulu m'en dire le prix, permettez moi de vous offrir cette petite piece d'argenterie comme un temoignage de ma reconnoissance, et recevez l'expression de toute celle que je reconnois vous devoir pour la parfaite guérison qui a été la suite de la cure que vous m'avêz fait suivre. Je vous aï dit, Monsieur, en quittant Brighton au mois d'Octobre dernier, que si mon hiver se passoit sans que j'éprouvasse aucun ressentiment ni du tic douloureux dont je souffrois depuis plus de 18 mois, ni des rhumatismes dont j'étois tourmentée depuis plusieurs années, je m'empresserois de vous écrire pour vous informer du plein succes de vos soins. Je remplis aujourd'hui cet engagement en vous ecrivant la présente, à la quelle je vous permets de donner toute publicité, et par laquelle je certifie que j'ai été complettement guérie par suite de la cure que vous m'avez administrée. Adieu, Monsieur, recevez l'assurance de ma plus parfaite estime.

La Comtesse TYSZKIEWICZ,
Princesse PONIATOWSKA.

[Translation.]

Paris, April 6th, 1825.

Sir,—I begin by thanking you for the small vial of oil which accompanied your letter of the 15th of March, and beg that as soon as you have received the parcel you expect from India, you will, according to your promise, send me a small stock of your oil, I mean the stronger of the two sorts. As you never would mention the price, allow me to present you with this small piece of plate as a token of my gratitude, which I feel myself bound in duty to acknowledge, for my perfect recovery in consequence of the treatment you prescribed. I told you, Sir, on my leaving Brighton in the month of October last, that if the winter passed without my feeling any return either of the *tic douloureux* with which I had been afflicted for more than 18 months, or of the rheumatism which had tormented me for many years, I would hasten to apprise you of the complete success of your attentions. I now fulfil my engagement by writing the present to you, to which I give you leave to give full publicity, and by which I certify, that I have been completely cured by the remedies you have administered to me. Farewell, Sir; receive the assurance of my most perfect esteem.

La Comtesse TYSZKIEWICZ,
Princesse PONIATOWSKA.

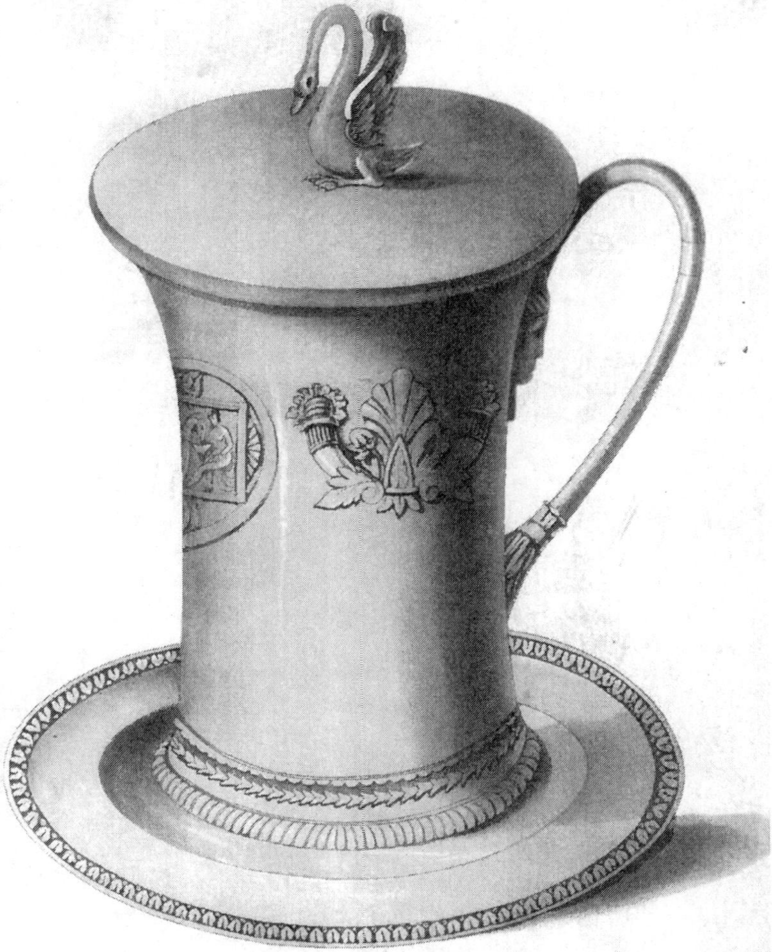

Representation
(of a)
SILVER CUP COVER AND DISH
PRESENTED TO
SAKE DEEN MAHOMED
by
H. S. H. The Princess Poniatowsky of Poland.

CASE XXV.

CASE OF SCIATICA.

Brighton, April 16, 1825.

Dear Sir,—I am happy to leave my testimony with you of the benefit I have received from the application of your Medicated Vapour Baths. When I arrived in Brighton last Monday week, I could with difficulty place my legs to the ground; I can now walk about without assistance either from stick or crutches. The Sciatica was my complaint. I sincerely trust I shall feel no more of it.

I have also derived benefit from your Indian Medicine.

Wishing you and your family your health,

I am, yours, obediently,

JAMES HOOD.

CASE XXVI.

CONTRACTION OF THE KNEE AND INFLAMMATION.

Mr. H. Weld has great pleasure in acknowledging the wonderful efficacy of Mr. Mahomed's Baths, in removing a very severe and obstinate inflammation of the knee, with which Mrs. H. Weld had been afflicted for more than a year and a half, and which had resisted all the usual remedies. When first she consulted Mr. Mahomed, the complaint was rapidly gaining ground, the limb was much contracted, and Mrs. Weld's strength was exhausted. The very first Bath afforded relief, and appeared to destroy all tendency to inflammation, as she never after experienced any return of it, though she immediately entered upon a more nourishing plan of diet. By perseverance in the use of the Vapour Baths and other of Mr. Mahomed's remedies, for nearly three months, Mrs. Weld was gradually restored to health and the perfect use of her limb, so much so, that she is now enabled to walk two hours together without fatigue. Mr. Mahomed is at liberty to make what use he pleases of this letter, as it is the united wish of Mr. and Mrs. Weld to promote his interest to the utmost of their power.

Chidcock House, June 4, 1825.

CASE XXVII.

CASE OF PALPITATION OF THE HEART AND COMPLICATED DISEASE.

TO MR. SAKE DEEN MAHOMED.

Dear Sir,—Although I have been incessant in recommending the valuable efficacy of your Medicated Vapour Baths since I myself experienced their effects, if you think any written statement of my case likely to benefit others, and serve you, I will most readily give it you.

In April, 1823, I was advised by a private friend to try your Baths, and place myself under your entire treatment, being then in a very nervous, low, debilitated state, subject to violent palpitation of the heart, tendency of blood to the head, dieted upon vegetables and water, and altogether quite ill. This indisposition I had been under near three years, brought on by domestic affliction and other connected causes, till it finally reduced me to an alarming illness in 1821-22, and the ultimate recovery from which (under the most eminent of the faculty) left me as herein described in April, 1823.

When urged by my friend to try your Baths, I quite ridiculed the idea as inapplicable to my case, and I believe nothing but the conviction that every expedient I had resorted to had failed, would finally have overcome my prejudice. Thus reluctantly did I submit to the use of the Vapour Baths: the first I took did me great service, aiding appetite, sleep, and digestion, quelling nervous excitement, and causing better circulation, without any of the alarming consequences I had apprehended; and a repetition of them for one fortnight, aided by your medicinal treatment, returned me to London the astonishment of every friend; and an occasional perseverance in them soon after, renovated me to my wonted health. Another remarkable instance of their peculiar efficacy in cases of languid circulation, occurred to me in March, 1824, when in London. I caught a severe inflammatory cold, which brought on my old symptoms, and required the use of digitalis and other baneful medicines, and left me very weak. As soon as able I went to Brighton for a Bath, and such was the torpid state of circulation in me, that with the vapour at 110 by the thermometer inside the Bath, I absolutely shivered, and had hot oils applied to restore it, which *no Warm Bath* could have done, neither could the heat have been *so* endured—one more Bath restored me to myself again. I am now quite well, but shall always resort to your Vapour Bath, whenever indisposed. I have finally no hesitation in saying that they have a pre-eminent claim to any Warm Bath, and may be used with success in most cases, but in almost any without the least apprehension, from the various diseases I have witnessed a recovery from by my own recommendation; whilst in all cases of contraction, rheumatic and other pains, I hesitate not, to pronounce them superior to any other treatment, from having been an eye witness to such recoveries as I could not otherwise have credited.

I remain, dear Sir,
Your constant well wisher,
HENRY POUNSETT.

Bartholomew-lane, London.
July, 1825.

CASE XXVIII.

TO MR. MAHOMED.

CASE OF RHEUMATIC AFFECTION.

Sir,—Having received a perfect cure from the use of your Vapour Baths, and thinking that a knowledge of the circumstance might be beneficial to those who may be afflicted as I have been, I will give a brief statement of the case and leave it to your discretion, whether or not to give it publicity. I was a great sufferer from extreme pain in my left side for some months, and was at length, obliged to leave my place of servitude and return home to my mother, who is a widow, and but ill able to provide for herself. I received every attention from an eminent medical gentleman, who at last candidly assured me, that he had done all he could, but recommended me to apply to a physician, which I did, but his prescriptions were of no use. I remained for five months without the least hope of ever again being able to get my living, when my late mistress proposed calling with me to consult you, as every other means had been resorted to without affording any permanent relief; but from the trial of your Vapour Baths for three weeks, I am perfectly restored to health,—am entirely free from the rheumatic affection which had seized the whole of my left side, and am now, consequently, able to take another situation. I know not how to express the gratitude I feel for the great act of humanity and generosity shewn me, as well as for the kindness and attentions of Mrs. Mahomed and attendants, having no remuneration to offer but my most gtateful acknowledgment.

I am authorised by my late mistress, Mrs. Fuller, of South-street, Lewes, to say, that any reference may be made to her, and she will be happy to give any further information that may be required; for such an entire cure far exceeded her most sanguine expectations.

I am, Sir,

Your's much indebted and obliged,

MARY ADE.

Hamsey,
Sept. 5, 1825.

CASE XXIX.

CASE OF PARALYSIS.

TO S. D. MAHOMED.

Sir,—I cannot in justice to you quit Brighton after five weeks' residence, without expressing the high gratification of acknowledging the great benefit I have experienced under your directions. I have been affected for nearly three years past with a partial paralytic affection of the left knee, extending to the ankle and foot, which by the use of the Vapour Bath and Shampooing is very much relieved, and I entertain no doubt but that I shall ultimately totally recover the perfect use of my limb.

JOHN ROSE, Surgeon,
Eye, Suffolk.

Sept. 27, 1825.

CASE XXX.

CASE OF LAMENESS.

Case of Miss Caroline Payne Gallway.—About three years ago she was attacked with a pain in her right foot, the cause of which could not be accounted for ; this pain continued increasing for twelve months, but only occasionally prevented her taking her usual exercise. On her return to England in the summer of 1823, it became so much worse that she was quite unable to walk without considerable pain, and her general health was affected. She went up to town, and remained there three weeks under the care of an eminent physician and surgeon ; the latter afterwards prescribed for her on her return into the country, but without the least relief ; the complaint continued increasing for eighteen months, during which time she consulted many other physicians and surgeons without the least benefit ; for the last six months she was unable to walk or put her foot to the ground, and even latterly to bear the motion of a carriage without great pain, and confined to her sofa. In the month of August, 1825, she came to Brighton to try the effects of Mahomed's Vapour Baths; after the fourth Bath she was able to walk without her stick, and at the end of six weeks perfectly recovered the use of her foot, and enabled to take her exercise as before the attack, and to walk for two hours or more at a time, without pain or inconvenience.

CASE XXXI.

CASE OF LAMENESS OF THE KNEE.

Sir,—I should hold myself greatly deficient in gratitude towards you, were I to think of quitting Brighton without leaving my acknowledgment of the great benefit I have received from the use of your Vapour and Shampooing Bath; and as it may possibly be of some public service, I beg to state that in consequence of a blow which I received on the knee by being accidentally thrown out of a chaise about fourteen months ago, an accumulation (as I am professionally informed) of the synovia had taken place underneath the knee, forming an enlarged bursa, but of such slow accumulation was it, that I did not experience any inconvenience until eight months after the accident, and then it increased so much as almost to prevent the possibility of walking. I have since that time been under the care of some of the most experienced gentlemen in the medical profession, by whose direction I have used various embrocations, pressure, and have repeatedly applied strong blister, in order to its dispersion, without success, but which I feared would terminate with a stiff joint or contracted leg, and was at last recommended by one of the most eminent practical surgeons of the present day, to try the effect of your Medicated Vapour Bath, and which, I am happy to say, in the course of a fortnight completely restored the free use of my leg, and I now walk perfectly easy with a very trifling sensation of pain indeed; and I am so satisfied of the benefit I have received, that I shall have pleasure in giving any information on the subject to any person whom you may think fit, or have occasion to refer to me.

I am, Sir,
Very faithfully yours,
W. ROUSSEAU.

Chertsey, Surrey, Sept. 28, 1825.

To Mr. Mahomed, Shampooing Surgeon, Brighton.

CASE XXXII.

CASE OF CONTRACTION ARISING FROM SPRAIN.

Miss Walker has great pleasure in acknowledging the benefit she has derived from Mr. Mahomed's Vapour Baths, in the case of a contraction arising from a sprain.

Tilehurst, Sept. 29, 1825.

CASE XXXIII.

CASE OF SPRAINED SHOULDER WITH STIFFNESS.

Stanmer, October 5, 1825.

Sir,—I have much pleasure in acknowledging the benefit which I derived from the use of your Vapour Bath. Early in the summer of 1823 I sprained my shoulder, which produced a stiffness (attended occasionally with pain) that in the course of time prevented my raising my arms to my head; at the beginning of the following autumn, I had recourse to your

Baths, which soon afforded the greatest relief, and ultimately restored the free use of my arm.

I am, Sir, &c. &c. &c.

M. CHICHESTER.

CASE XXXIV.

CASE OF PARALYSIS.

Miss Gordon was attacked in the summer of 1824, with a bilious fever, attended with determination of blood to the head. When recovering from this, an error in diet brought on a relapse, when she was seized with paralysis of the lower extremities. She came to Brighton in April, 1825, perfectly unable to stand, and began the use of the Vapour Bath and Shampooing daily. From this time her improvement was most rapid, and in the following September she was able to walk across the room without assistance, and to walk a mile merely leaning upon a person's arm. Miss Gordon has much pleasure in bearing this public testimony to the great benefit she has derived from Mr. Mahomed's Medicated Vapour Bath.

November 3, 1825.

CASE XXXV.

CASE OF LAMENESS IN THE KNEE.

TO MR. MAHOMED.

No. 1, St. Dunstan's Hill, London.
Nov. 9, 1825.

SIR,—I have much pleasure in recording the great and speedy benefit derived from your Indian Medicated Vapour Baths and Shampooing system.

I suffered severe lameness in the knee from the effects of a cold, and was unable to walk without the aid of a crutch, for nearly two months, during which period I received little or no relief from a variety of appropriate outward applications: I then subjected myself to your Vapour Baths,—three of which mitigated, and sixteen entirely removed the evil above described.

I remain, Sir,

Your obliged servant,

CHARLES SKIPPER.

CASE XXXVI.

CASE OF LAMENESS.

Mrs. E. Lamb's compliments to Mr Mahomed, has returned the crutches, and begs Mr. M. to accept her best thanks by leaving them as a proof of the benefit she has derived from his Vapour Baths.

Ship-street Gardens, Brighton, Nov. 15, 1825,
Or No. 1, Terrace, Kensington.

CASE XXXVII.

CASE OF LUMBAGO.

DEAR SIR,—Although amongst the majority of formidable cases, wherein your superior mode of Indian Shampooing and application of Medicated Vapour Baths to the alleviation of human afflictions, (of which abundant proofs are extant), mine must appear of very minor importance in the scale of comparison; candour compels me to declare, in grateful return for your attention and ability, that *they were not so considered by me*, while suffering at various times under the pain of lumbago, stiff-neck, and rheumatism, each local attack, at distant intervals, having been happily dissipated by your soothing and pleasant system; by which, although previously ill at ease, I was as suddenly and completely restored, as if I had never been affected. Thinking the knowledge of these restorations may be as beneficial to others, as they have been pleasant to myself, you are at liberty to make what use you please of the sentiments of

Your obliged, humble servant,
C. BEW,

Nov. 17th, 1825. East-street, Brighton.
To S. D. Mahomed, Indian Vapour Bath.

CASE XXXVIII.

CASE OF SCROFULA AND LAMENESS.

Brighton, Nov. 20, 1825.

SIR,—The great benefit my son has derived from your Vapour Bath has induced me to make his case known to the public: he was from his birth a very fine healthy child until he was two years old, when he caught the meazles, which left him in a very bad state, full of scrofulous humour all over him, with a swelling on his knee. I had every advice I possibly could have, but he still continued getting worse both in bodily health and lameness, his leg becoming very much contracted; in short, his knee was so alarming, that I was persuaded by a medical man to allow him to suffer amputation above the knee, as the only chance of saving his life. As a last resource, I was induced to try your Vapour Bath, and I must say, with little hopes of success on my part, as the child at that time was a mere skeleton, nearly blind with one eye, and in a most shocking state, with loss of appetite, and could not move across the room without the use of crutches. To my great surprise, after taking three or four of the Vapour Baths, his appetite began to increase, and he continued getting better. After about two months he left off his crutches and walked with a stick, and in respect of his bodily health, no child could be better, and so he continues, free from all humour in his body and the picture of health, to the astonishment of every one who knew him. I feel it a duty incumbent on me, to return you my grateful thanks for restoring my child to the state he is now in, and I shall always pray for your welfare. Any person wishing to see the child, I shall feel it a great pleasure to give them every information I can on the subject.

I have also to return you my grateful thanks for the cure you have made of my eldest son, whom I sent to you with a dreadful swelled knee, occasioned by a fall, so bad that he could not get in and out of the fly without great assistance. I am happy to say, that after taking three of the Vapour Baths, he was enabled to walk home without assistance, and is now quite recovered.

By publishing this in your book, you will much oblige,

Sir, your most obedient,

and ever grateful servant,

DANIEL LUCAS.

No. 5, Edward-street, Brighton.

To Mr. Mahomed.

CASE XXXIX.

CASE OF SCROFULA AND CONTRACTION OF THE KNEE.

Brighton, November 29th, 1825.

DEAR SIR,—My younger sister residing in Hanover, having been for upwards of six years afflicted with a contraction and swelling in the knee, evidently of scrofulous origin, which had baffled the utmost efforts of her medical advisers, and after the most powerful stimulants, such as perpetual blisters and even the burning iron, had been applied in vain; I was induced to send for her over, in order to try whether the Vapour Bath and Shampooing might be of benefit to her. On her arrival she was in the most emaciated state, her complexion pale, and hardly able to move with crutches; after a dozen of your Vapour Baths, she shewed symptoms of improvement, and by continuing the same for upwards of six months, she was so much restored as to be able to walk without crutch or stick a couple of miles; and by using the cold sea bath afterwards for six months, she returned to her parents in Germany in such an improved state of health, that her friends could hardly recognise her. My father in his letter to me, most feelingly said, "Having convinced myself that I again beheld my child, I went on my knees to thank the Almighty for her wonderful restoration." Two years and a half having now elapsed since her return, I am happy to inform you that she is now in the same improved state as when she left England.

I am, my dear Sir,

Yours truly,

C. KRAMER.

TO SAKE DEEN MAHOMED

SHAMPOOING SURGEON,

BRIGHTON.

Herald of health ! whose spells of charmed pow'r
Soothe the deep anguish of affliction's hour,
Assuage, with healing art, the pangs of grief,
And on the pain-worn suff'rer pour relief,
Steep the rack'd sense in balm of sweetest sleep,
And close the eyes that only wak'd to weep ;
Bid Sorrow's woes, Affection's trials cease,
And in the ear of Anguish whisper " Peace."—

O let thy volume spread thy well-earn'd fame,
That distant vot'ries now may bless thy name,
And seek, from thee, our nature's dearest wealth,
Our God's best blessing, the sweet boon of health !

R.

Brighton, 1st December, 1825.

CHAP. VIII.

The following names are submitted to the Public, in further testimony of approval of the Baths under my direction. They are principally the names of Subscribers since the year 1820, most of whom have experienced the benefits of the *Vapour Baths and Shampooing*, either medicinally, as a restorative from fatigue, or, perhaps, more generally speaking, as a luxury, taken in lieu of the common Water Bath. The list comprises, however, but a very small portion of the names which are actually to be found in my Subscription book, and which I have omitted to transcribe in this place, from a wish not to swell out the book to an unnecessary length.

Arran, Earl of.
Alvanley, Lord.
Ashbrook, Viscountess
Antrobus, Sir E.
Afflesh, Gen. Sir James.
Affiesh, Lady,
Amon, Col.
Armstrong, Col.
Abbott, Mr. 3, Leicester-place, London.
Abbott, Mrs. 3, Leicester-square, London
Abbott, Mr. Llandberre Hall, Denbigh.
Abbott, Mr. P. H.
Abbott, Mr. James, Hanwell, Essex.
Abingdon, Mr. John
Abingdon, Mr.
Abraham, Mr. I. Isle of Wight.
Ackermann, Mr.
Ackington, Mrs. 6, East-cliff.

Adair, Mr. Minories, London.
Adam, Mr. A. London.
Adams, Miss 15, Regency-square.
Adams, Mr. S. Ware.
Adams, Mr. R.
Ading, Mr. Plaistow, Essex.
Ailes, Mr. T.
Aley, Mrs. 4, German-place.
Alcock, Mr. 21, New Steine.
Allen, Mr. London.
Allen, Mrs. Marine-parade.
Allen, Mr. J. W. Pulteney-street, Bath.
Allever, Mr. Shoreham.
Allister, Mrs. 46, East-cliff.
Anderson, Mr. W.
Anderson, Mr.
Anandon, Mrs. John, 73, King's-road.
Anwyl, Mr. Ellis, Five-field Chase.
Antwesdel, Mr. J.
Apsland, Mrs.
Appold, Mrs. 22, East-cliff.
Armstrong, Mr. C. Croydon.
Arthur, Mr. London.
Archer, Mr. John, Saffron Walden, Essex.
Ashburner, Mr. Birmingham.
Ashly, Mr. J. Adelphi-terrace.
Ashness, Mr. London.
Ashby, Mr.
Ashby, Mrs. T.
Atkinson, Mr. J.
Atkinson, Mr. Hampstead, Middlesex.
Atkinson, Mr. I. Northampton.
Aveling, Mr. Brewery, Spitalfields.
Austin, Mr. W.
Austin, Rev. I. Oakham, Surrey.
Avarne, Mr. London.

Ayton, Mr. I. Eccles Hall, Norfolk.
Aytoun, Mr. James.

Bayning, Lord, 9, Bedford-square.
Blachford, Lady Isabella.
Berkeley, Lady, Emily.
Beresford, Lord.
Beresford, Sir John.
Beresford, Sir M.
Beresford, Miss.
Beauchamp, Earl of.
Bolingbroke, Lord.
Byland, Countess, 44, Church-street.
Byland, Count Col. Blackheath, Kent.
Berconby, Hon. Mrs.
Bentinck, Lord Charles.
Backhouse, Major Gen.
Bateman, Major-Gen.
Blunt, Major-Gen.
Brown, Lieut. Col.
Burgoyne, Sir John.
Burgoyne, Mr. Montague.
Burgoyne, Mr. Fred.
Burney, Rev. Dr.
Blackman, Dr.
Brett, Rev. George, Ranelagh, London.
Betts, Rev. Mr. T. D. Wortham.
Burford, Rev. Mr. 4, West-cliff.
Baker, Capt. R. N.
Barclay, Capt.
Bankes, Hon. Mrs.
Barnard, Sir A. F.
Barnard, Lady.
Bowater, Adm. Princes-street, Pavilion-parade.
Branford, Capt. R. N.
Bellasis, Mrs. Col.

Ball, Miss, 41, Marlboro'-place.
Babington, Mrs.
Bailey, Miss
Bailey, Mr. 5, Phœnix-street, Somers-town.
Bailey, Mr. London.
Baillie, Mr. J. Western-house.
Baird, Miss, Piccadilly.
Baker, Mr. Thomas, Hemsted, Herts.
Baldwin, Mr. J. Cannon-street, London.
Banbury, Mrs. Russell-house.
Bannister, Mrs. C.
Bannister, Mr. G.
Banner, Mr. F. G. 36, Marine-parade.
Bannandan, Mr. York-hotel.
Barclay, Miss, 7, East-cliff.
Barclay, Mr. R. Regency-square.
Bardeline, Mr. S. Bucks.
Barlow, Mr. R. P. London.
Barnard, Mr. W. Euston-square, London.
Barnard, Mrs.
Barnard, Lieut. Geo. R.N. Bellevue Cottage.
Barnes, Mrs.
Barnet, Mrs.
Barrett, Miss.
Barry, Mrs.
Barry, Mr.
Barry, Mr. E. West-square.
Barry, Mr. T. Newington-causeway.
Barton, Mr. Croydon.
Barham, Mr.
Barker, Mr. S. Gates's Boarding-house.
Bates, Dr.
Baxter, Mr. W. Bellevue-lodge, Reigate.
Baxter, Mr. London.
Bayham, Mr. 7, Upper Grenville-place.
Baylis, Mr. W.

Bayford, Mr.
Beard, Mr.
Beaufort, Mr.
Beaumont, Mrs. R. 6, King's-road.
Beckett, Mr.
Beech, Mr. Chelsea.
Belcher, Mrs. 24, Steine.
Bell, Mrs.
Bell, Miss
Belstead, Mr.
Bennet, Mr. J. S.
Benton, Mr. Change-alley, London.
Benton, Mr. G.
Bensusan, Mr. A. L. Great Prescott-street.
Benyon, Mr.
Berkeley, Mrs.
Bernard, Miss
Bernard, Mr. London.
Berger, Mrs: S.
Bernett, Mr. G. B.
Best, Mr.
Bethell, Mr.
Bethell, Mrs. 20, Marine-parade.
Beulle, Mr.
Bicknell, Mr. Rob.
Biddle, Mr. A.E. High Wycomb, Berks.
Biddulph, Miss, Crescent-lodge.
Biggers, Mr. R.
Biggs, Mr. Matt. Newtimber.
Billing, Mr. R. Reading, Berks.
Bine, Mr.
Bingley, Mr. B. London.
Bishop, Mrs. 41, Old-steine.
Bishop, Mr. Jas.
Bishop, Major H.
Black, Miss, Grand-parade.

Blake, Mr. Jermyn-street, St. James's, London
Blacket, Mr. 51, King's-road.
Blacket, Mrs.
Blann, Mr.
Blayds, Mr.
Bland, Mr. 62, Grand-parade.
Blackstock, Mr.
Blackwell, Miss E.
Blackenhagen, Miss E.
Blew, Mr. Worcester.
Blew, Mr. jun. ditto.
Blew, Mr. E.
Blew, Mr. R. jun:
Blencowe, Mr. 23, Steine.
Boehm, Mr.
Bodfield, Mr.
Bodfield, Mrs.
Bolougne, Miss.
Bonhar, Mr. J. H.
Boniface, Miss, Drayton, Sussex.
Boniface, Mr. Drayton, Sussex.
Bonnett, Mr. T.
Boon, Miss, King's-road.
Booth, Mr. F. Russell-square.
Booth, Mr. P. York-hotel.
Booth, Mr. Felix, ditto.
Booth, Mr. Coventry.
Bolton, Mr. Great Queen-street, Lincoln's-Inn-fields, London.
Bone, Mr. R. Ockham.
Bond, Mr. J. Ipswich.
Bonner, Miss, Guildford.
Bonar, Mrs. 49, Regency-square.
Borel, Mons. de Fauche, 33, Haymarket, London.
Bornce, Mrs. 9, Gardner-street.
Borough, Miss.
Borry, Mrs.

Boswell, Mr. London.
Bott, Mr. Nantwich.
Botting, Mr. G. Lewes.
Bovell, Mr. J. R.
Bowden, Mr. Queen's Royals.
Bowden, Mr. London.
Bowderry, Mrs.
Bowdoin, Mr. T.
Bowles, Miss.
Bowles, Mr. J. Middleton-house, Enfield.
Boulnois, Mr. Tower, London.
Boys, Mr. John.
Boys, Mr. Josh.
Bourn, Mr. J.
Brasier, Mr. Westfield Lodge.
Bravo, Mr. A.
Bradburne, Mr. Marine-mansion:
Bradley, Mrs. R. 42, King's-road.
Brandram, Mr. W.
Branton, Miss, 47, King's-road.
Bredel, A. 19, Wormwood-street, or Lloyd's.
Brent, Mr. York-hotel.
Bridges, Mr.
Briggs, Miss.
Brichton, Mr. G. Hornsey.
Brinton, Mr. J. Portsmouth.
Bridge, Mr. Thos. Buttebury, Essex.
Bridges, Mr. 20, Steine.
Brinchley, Mr. J. Gravesend, Kent.
Bridell, Mr. Devonshire-place.
Broadbent, Miss.
Broadwood, Mr. H.
Brooks, Mr. G. Lisson-grove.
Brooksbank, Mr. Lower Grosvenor-street.
Bromhead, Mr. Lincoln.
Brown, Miss, Laughton, Sussex.

Brown, Mr. Carter, United States of America.
Browne, Mr. T. Simmon's-Inn, London.
Browne, Miss, 30, West-cliff.
Browne, Mrs, 52, Steine.
Browne, Mr. ditto.
Brunton, Mr. John.
Buck, Miss.
Buck, Mrs. 40, King's-road.
Buckingham, Mr. J. S. Marine-hotel.
Buck, Mr. Birmingham.
Bulbeck, Mr. John, Havant.
Bull, Mr.
Buller, Mr. J.
Bullivant, Mrs.
Bullivant, Mr.
Bullock, Mr.
Bunt, Mrs, Guildford.
Burford, Rev. Mr., 4, West-cliff.
Burke, Mr. London.
Burncan, Mrs. Old Steine.
Burnett, Mr. J.
Burnett, Mr. J. F., Bedford-hill, Tooting.
Burnett, Mr. H., London.
Burr, Mr. Robert, Chatham.
Burrell, Miss, East-lodge.
Burry, Mr. H.
Burry, Mr. German-place.
Burrell, Mr. W. Watford, Herts.
Burrough, Miss G. West-cliff-house.
Burroughs, Miss.
Burls, Mr. East-cliff.
Burras, Mr. James, London.
Burrows, Mr. S. Hackney.
Butchell, Mr. E. Van, 24, Broad-street, Golden-square, London.
Bntcher, Mrs.
Butler, Mr. J. Cheam, Surry.

Butterworth, Mr. John, Long-lane, Southwark.
Byrne, Miss, 29, New Steine.
Bye, Mr, London.
Buzzard, Mr. Thomas, Jewry-street, Aldgate.

Chichester, Countess of,
Chichester, Earl of,
Conyngham, Marquis of,
Conyngham, Lady M.,
Conyngham, Lady E.,
Conyngham, Lord F.,
Clanwilliam, Lord.
Cockburn, Lady,
Codrington, Lady.
Constable, Lady, 33, Regency-square.
Constable, Miss, Isabella.
Calthorpe, Lady.
Cole, Lady Elizabeth.
Cornwallis, Marchioness of,
Cornwallis, Lady Mary.
Cornwallis, Lady Louisa.
Cornwallis, Lady I.
Copley, Sir J.
Copley, Lady, 12, Regency-square.
Compton, Sir John.
Carpenter, Hon. Mrs.
Carpenter, Major.
Coffin, Admiral Sir I.
Cholmondeley, Mr. F.
Colpoys, Griffith, Vice-admiral.
Cullum, Sir Thomas, Bart.
Craufurd, Major, Royal Lancers.
Calvert, Capt., Grenadier-guards.
Cadogan, Capt. 34, Regency-square.
Capel, Gen. Marine-hotel.
Cuppas, Major Gen.

Coghlan, Gen.
Cooke, Col.
Chatfield, Capt. A. S.
Clifford, Capt.
Clayton, Rev. Mr. John.
Capper, Rev. Mr. James.
Chester, Rev. Mr. Rob.
Campbell, Rev. Mr. H., Minchinhampton.
Chapman, Rev. W. H.
Chappell, Lieut. R. N.
Calvert, Mr. E.
Campbell, Mr.
Campbell, Mr.
Campbell, Mr. G.
Campernowne, Mr. Cricklade, Wilts.
Canning, Miss.
Capper, Mrs.
Carnday, Mr. J. W:
Carter, Mr. J. C., Norwich.
Carter, Mrs.
Carter, Capt. R. W.
Cater, Mr.
Catlin, Mr. N. Saffron Walden.
Cattley, Miss.
Cartwright, Mr.
Canty, Mr.
Cazenove, Mr. Crouch-end, Hornsey.
Chalk, Mr.
Chalkley, Mr. R.
Chambre, Miss, New-steine hotel.
Chapman, Mr. E. Castle-square.
Chapman, Mr. Robt. 34, Marine-parade.
Charlesworth, Mr. S. 21, Devonshire-place, London.
Charlton, Mr. L.
Charman, Mr. F.
Charrote, Mr. St. Paul's Church-yard.

Chatfield, Mrs., London.
Chatham, Mr. R. Holborn, London.
Chesshyre, Miss.
Cherrill, Mr. E. London.
Cherrill, Miss, 44, Marine-parade.
Child, S. P. Hackney.
Child, Mr. Huntingdon.
Child, Mr. C. Horsham.
Chipperfield, Mr. E. T.
Chitty, Mr. Lewes.
Christian, Mrs. Henry, 29, Newman-street.
Christie, Mr.
Clapton, Mrs.
Clapton, Mr. Kennington-common.
Clark, Mr. London.
Clark, Miss, Paragon House, Brighton.
Clark, Mr. John.
Cleaver, Mr. J. Kennington-common.
Clementson, Mrs. 9, Western-place.
Clissold, Mr. Gloucester
Cobb, Mr.
Cockburn, Mr. Best's Boarding-house.
Cocksedge, Mr. Bury St. Edmund's.
Cohen, Mrs. 13, Bedford-square.
Cohen, Mr. H. A. Brixton, Surry.
Cohen, Mr. J. H. 23, St. James's-street.
Colbatch, Mr. E. 159, Minories.
Collins, Mrs. Laytonstone, Essex.
Collins, Mr. Sunbury.
Collings, Mr.
Colquhoun, Mr. 13, Broad-street.
Colebroke, Miss, 10, Bedford-square.
Collman, Mr. L.
Colvill, Mr.
Comber, Mr. W.
Connor, Mr. N.

Conry, Mrs. 16, Regency-square.
Cookburn, Mr. Ship-street.
Cook, Mr. G. S.
Cooper, Mr. B. Royal Exchange Assurance, London.
Cooper, Mr. F. 10, Cannon-place.
Cooper, Mr. B. Chancery-lane, London.
Cooper, Mr. F. Windsor.
Copland, Mr. Chas.
Copeland, Mrs.
Coppinger, Mr. Devonshire-square, London.
Courtoy, Mrs. 26, Lower-rock-gardens.
Cowley, Miss.
Cowley, Mr.
Cowley, Mr. S. N.
Cox, Mrs. 13, West Cliff.
Cox, Mr. J. P.
Cox, Mr. Francis, West-street, Brompton.
Cox, Mr. J. P. Inner Temple, London.
Cox, Mr. Chichester.
Cox, Mr. John.
Cripps, John.
Critchett, Mr. R.
Crocraft, Mr. Montague-square, London.
Cronfood, Mrs. C. 98, West-cliff.
Crosby, Mrs. and family.
Crosman, Mr. J.
Crowder, Mr.
Crowley, Mr. A.
Crump, Mrs. 2, Marine-parade.
Cubitt, Mr. W.
Cuff, Miss.
Cule, Mrs. 27, Broad-street.
Cullen, Miss, 6, Bedford-square.
Cumine, Mr. J. King-street, Borough, London.
Curle, Mr. W. Pimlico.
Currie, Mr. Francis Gore, East Horsley Park, Surry.

Currie, Mr. Raikes, 33, Wimpole-street, London.
Cutbrush, Mr. Robert, Maidstone.
Cymber, Mr. H. London.
Curtis, D. Cowley, Middlesex.
Curzon, Mr.

Devonshire, his Grace the Duke of.
Douglas, Marquis of.
Dewes, Lord.
Dallas, Sir Geo.
Dallas, Capt.
Dawkins, Capt.
Denby, Col. W. Percy-street, London.
Denny, Lady.
Dolben, Sir English, Northampton.
Dormer, Lady Ann.
Doyle, General, Sir Charles.
Duncan, Mr. J. Trinity College, Cambridge.
Dyke, Sir Thos. Lullingtone-castle, Kent.
Dawson, Lady Louisa.
Douglas, Admiral, J. E.
Dacre, Lieut.-Col.
Danvers, Mr. B.
Dangerfield, Mr.
Dangerfield, Mrs.
Dangerfield, Mr. T.
Dalton, Mr.
Davidson, Mr. Chas.
Davie, Mr. Peckham.
Davis, Mr. John, Machyntteth, Montgomeryshire.
Davy, Mr. Bedford-square.
Dawes, Mr. Rye, Sussex.
Day, George, London.
Day, Mrs. Thos. Maidstone.
Deane, Mr. West-cliff Lodge.
Davenport, Mr. Lime-street, London.

De Bath, Major.
Dear, Mr. F. C.
Delesert, Mr. A. a native of Switzerland, living in Paris.
Denham, Mr. James.
Denman, Miss M.
Dering, Mr.
Detvityick, C. V. Mr. from Antwerp.
Despons, Mr. 41, King's-road.
Deval, Mr. R. Buckingham-street, Fiztroy-square :
Devereux, Mr. London.
De Beauvoir, Mr. Benyon, 75, Marine-parade.
De Wints, Gen. Count, 15, King's-road.
Davis, Mr. Corbet-court, London.
De Lisle, Stoke-Newington.
Devis, Mr. H. Stoke-Newington,
De Gullon, Mr. P. E.
Dickins, Mr. John.
Dickenson, Mr.
Dickens, Mr. Chas. Scrase.
Dingle, Mr. W.
Dickenson, Mr. T. P.
Dodfrey, Mr. John, Highgate,
Donat, Mr. J. A. 11, Pavilion-parade.
Dorset, Mrs. 75, West-street.
Doveton, Col.
Douglas, Mr. 18th Regiment.
Down, Mr. E. London.
Downess, Mrs.
Downing, Mrs. E.
Dowsland, Mr. W. 47, Marine-parade.
Dowding, Mr. 61, Marine-parade.
Downs, Mr. J. Hertford.
Doyle, Mr. Camomile-street.
Driver, Mr. E. New Bridge-street.
Druruod, Mr.
Dredge, Mr.

Doyson, Mr.
Drewitt, Mr. G. Peppering, Arundel.
Drysdale, Mr. H.
Drummond, Mr. John, Croydon.
Dunnage, Mrs. 70, Marine-parade.
Du Croz, Mr. S. Brook-street, London.
Dubois, Mr.
Duff, Mr.
Duke, Mr. John, Leominster.
Duke, H. Clapham, Surrey.
Duncan, Mr.
Duncan, Mr. 17th Lancers.
Dunn, Mrs.
Dunn, Mr. R. Threadneedle-street, London.
Dundas, Dr.
Duncomb, Mrs.
Dyson, Miss, 29, East-cliff.
Dyster, Mr. Leadenhall-street, London.
Dysart, Mr.

Essex, Countess of, 6, Pavilion-parade.
Elphinstone, Lord.
Edmonstone, Hon. Lady, 61, Marine-parade.
Exarque of Cyprus, Joannichios.
Exeter, Lord.
Eltose, Sir Abraham.
Eamer, Lieut. R. N.
Eamer, Mr. 4, Bedford-square.
Eaton, Mrs. East-cliff.
Eden, Miss.
Edgar, Mr. Piccadilly.
Eddie, Mr. J. A.
Edwards, Captain.
Edwards, Mrs. Marine-parade,
Edwards, Mr. Thos. Newport, Essex.
Edwards, Mr. 42, Conduit-street, Hanover-square, London.

Edwards, Mr. T. Paragon, Southwark.
Edmonds, Mr.
Egerton, Hon. Mrs. 9, Broad-street.
Eggington, Mr. Bilbroke, Staffordshire.
Elcho, Dowager Lady, 36, Marine-parade.
Ellis, Mr. C, 78, King's-road.
Ellis, Mr. J. D. London.
Elliot, Mr. Stafford.
Elwyn, Rev. Mr. Sandwich, Kent.
Elteen, Mr. Kensington.
Elley, Mr.
Emery, Mr. London.
Enfield, Mr. G.
Engleheart, Mr. H.
Entwistle, Mr.
Entwistle, Mr. Rushulme, Lancashire.
Espinasse, Col.
Etheridge, Mr.
Espinasse, Mr. R.
Evans, Miss.
Evans, Mr. N. B.
Evans, Mr. J. London.
Evans, Mr. 43, Grand-parade.
Everard, Rev. E.
Exeter, Mrs. 30, King's-road.
Eyre, Mr. 111, New Bond-street, London.

Falmouth, Viscountess.
Ford, Lady.
Frankland, Sir Thomas, Thirkleley, Yorkshire.
Falconer, Lieut. R. N.
French, Lieut.-Col.
French, Capt.
Fancourt, Rev. L.
Fairlie, Mr. Whoredon.
Farel, Mr. J. M. 10, Vine-street, London.

Fowke, Sir Frederick, Bart. Lowesby, Leicestershire.
Fayle, Mr. Clifton.
Fearon, Mr.
Feaves, Mr. L.
Fell, Mr. J. High-street, Borough.
Fennell, Mr. T.
Fenton, Miss.
Farquharson, Mrs. 78, Grand-parade.
Ferrers, Mr. T. B.
Ferron, Mrs.
Finch, Mrs. 26, East-cliff.
Finch, Mr.
Fisher, Mr.
Fisher, Mr. W. Highgate.
Fitzgerald, Dr. London.
Fitzgerald, Mr.
Fitzherbert, Mrs.
Fitzherbert, Mr. Blackdown, Sussex:
Fleming, Mr. London.
Fletcher, Mr. J. London.
Fletcher, Mr. R. Balsham, Cambridgeshire.
Fletcher, Rev. E.
Flint, Mr. Kingston, near Lewes.
Frampton, Mr. W.
Forbes, Mr.
Francis, Mr.
Francis, Rev. C.
Frankland, Mr. 77, Marine-parade.
Ford, Capt.
Ford, Mrs.
Foster, Mr.
Forster, Mr.
Forth, Mrs. 46, King's-road.
Forth, Miss.
Forth, Miss C.
Forth, Mr.

Forth, Mr. John, Luton.
Fowler, Rev. R. H.
Fox, Mr. 37, Marine-parade.
Francis, Mr.
Franks, Miss.
Frant, Miss, Gloucester-place.
Fraser, Mr. A. Bengal Medical Establishment.
Fraser, Capt. Woodcott-house, Oxon.
Freelove, Mr. W. Isleworth, Surry.
Freeman, Mrs.
Freeman, Mr. Thos. London.
Frinns, Mr. J. Dover.
Frisell, Mr. Paris.
Frith, Mrs. 35, Old Steine.
Frost, Miss.
Fry, Mr. London.
Fryer, Mr. T. Cambridge.
Fuller, Miss.
Fuller, Mr. J. 70, Grand-parade.
Fuller, Mr. Josh. Southover, Lewes
Furlonger, Mr. London,
Fuseli, Mrs.

Gallwey, Lady H. Payne.
Gower, Lord F. Levison
Garlies, Lord.
Grantly, Lord.
Grantly, Lady, Kier.
Grant, Sir William.
Gore, Lady, West-cliff House.
Gordon, Lady Jane.
Gordon, Hon. Mrs. Hallyburton.
Gordon, Sir W. Duff, Bart. 38, Lower Brook-street.
Gordon, Sir Jenison, Bart. 1, Bedford-street.
Gordon, Dr.
Gaillord, Miss.

Gairkes, Dr.
Gale, Mr.
Gale, Mr. J. Surgeon, Newington.
Gale, Mr. Surgeon, Alfred-place.
Gallup, Mr.
Garcia, Mr. A. R. Camden-place.
Garraway, Mr. Chelsea.
Garrett, Mr. Tower-street, London.
Gatty, Mr. Charter House.
Gatty, Mrs. 80, Grand-parade.
Gaullaret, Mr. Chas. Bryanston-square.
Gaviller, Mr.
Gawther, Mr.
George, Mrs.
George, Mr. Enfield.
George, Mr. J. 73, Holborn-bridge.
Gerring, Mr. W. Swindon, Wilts.
Gerring, Mr. C. Northfield, Farringdon, Berks.
Ghrimes, Mr. W. Ludgate, London.
Gibbon, Mrs. W.
Gibbons, Mrs. E. 13, North-street.
Gibson, Mr. J. R.
Gibson, Mr.
Gibson, Mr. R. G.
Gilbert, Mr. Long-acre, London.
Giles, Mr.
Gill, Mr.
Gill, Miss Augusta.
Gilbertson, Miss, 52, Judd-street, London.
Gillespie, Mr. America-square.
Gillibrand, Mr.
Ginger, Mrs. College-street.
Gillum, Dr.
Glenny, Miss. S. Barking, Essex.
Glover, Mr.
Godley, Mr. Geo. London.

Goddard, Mr. Seymour-street, London.
Goodall, Mr. 31, King's-road.
Godwin, Mr. J. H.
Godfrey, Rev. Mr. W.
Gooch, Mr.
Good, Mr. J. C.
Gordon, Mr. F.
Gore, Mr. R. H.
Gorringe, Mr. W. P.
Gowri, Sir F. L.
Graham, Capt.
Grant, Capt.
Grey, Lieut.-Col,
Green, Capt. R.N.
Gotobed, Mr.
Gould, Miss.
Gould, Mr. W.
Grant, Mr.
Grant, Mrs. W. B.
Grant, Mr. James.
Gray, Mr. W. Fleet-street, London.
Gray, Mr. R. Somerset-place, ditto.
Gray, Mr. R. A. Peckham-rye, Surry.
Graves, Mr. 28, Bedford-square.
Greenwood, Miss.
Gregg, Miss.
Gregory, Mr. T.
Green, Mr. Bedford.
Green, Mr. Gravely, Herts.
Gresson, Mr. 27, Steine.
Grevile, Mr. Algernon.
Greasly, Mr. T. T. Solicitor, Nottingham.
Greaves, Mr. 72, Marine-parade.
Griffin, Mr. W.
Griffith, Mrs. D. 56, Regency-square.
Griffith, Miss, Arundel.

Grimness, Mr. B. 10, Cannon-place.
Grinfield, Mr. West Drayton, Middlesex.
Grosvenor, Mr.
Gosseer, Mr. W. German-place.
Grilish, M. from St. Petersburgh.
Gower, Mr. W. 31, King's-road.
Guedalla, Mrs.
Gurney, Mr.
Gurney, Miss.
Gullyes, Mr. C. Stantones-wareff.

Harvey, Lady Sophia.
Hamilton, Duchess of.
Hamilton, Lord A.
Howard, Lord, of Effingham.
Harper, Lady.
Hartwell, Sir F. J.
Harley, the Ladies.
Hislop, Lieut.-Gen. Sir Thomas.
Hislop, Lady.
Hastings, Gen. Sir Charles.
Hepburn, Major-General.
Hesketh, Sir Thomas, Bart. Rufford-hall, Lancashire.
Hesketh, Mr.
Hughes, Lieut.-Col. James.
Hilton, Captain, King's-road.
Hamilton, Capt. A. P. Royal Navy, Marine-hotel.
Hodgson, Capt.
Howes, Capt. S. Marine-house.
Hooker, Rev. Dr.
Hunter, Dr.
Henderson, Mr. B. C. Surgeon.
Hewgill, Rev. Mr. F. 41, Steine.
Hodges, Rev. H. 10, East-cliff.
Hall, Rev. Thomas J. Waldon, Essex.
Howell, Rev. Mr.

Hack, Mr. W. Ware, Herts.
Hagger, Mr.
Hague, Miss, Tottenham.
Hall, Mrs. King's-road.
Hall, Mr. Leyton, Essex.
Halls, Mr. David, Bottleys, Surry.
Halman, Lieut. James, R.N.
Hallam, Mr. 4, King's-road.
Hamer, Mrs. Chester-place, Kennington.
Hamlet, Miss, Bloomsbury-place.
Hammond, Mr. I. Marine-hotel.
Hammond, Mr. Henry.
Hammond, Mr. Thomas, 3, Grafton-street.
Hamilton, Mr. Bedford-square.
Hammett, Mr. 9, Regency-square.
Hammersley, Mr. G. Devonshire-place.
Hamwell, Mrs. and Miss.
Hancock, Mr. and Miss E.
Hankey, Mr. James, 84, King's-road.
Hankey, Mr. A. Fenchurch-street, London.
Hand, Mr. T. Gower-street, London.
Hanwood, Mrs.
Hardcastle, Miss E.
Hardman, Mr. J. London.
Hardyman, Mrs. 27, Bedford-square.
Hardinge, Mrs. and Miss C. 57, Regency-square.
Harling, Mr. H. 3, Brewer-street, Bloomsbury.
Hargraves, Mr. Tunbridge Wells.
Harman, Mrs. Princes-street.
Harpur, Mr. Oxford.
Harris, Mr. W. London.
Harris, Mr. Brompton-crescent.
Harrison, Mrs. E.
Harrison, Mrs. 3, George-street, Manchester-square, London.
Harrison, Mr. Inner Temple.
Harrison, Mr. Lewis, 13, German-place.

Harrison, Mr. Edward, 9, Berkeley-street.
Harrison, Mr. John J. St. James's-street, London.
Harryet, Mr.
Hart, Mr. Norfolk-house.
Hart, Mr. W. Nelson-terrace, Stoke Newington.
Hart, Mr. Mecklenburgh-square, London.
Hartwell, Miss.
Hartwell, Mr. James, Uxbridge.
Hastings, Mr. F.
Haughton, Mrs. Dulwich.
Haughton, Mr.
Haultain, Mr. 28, Bedford-square.
Hawes, Mr. F.
Hawkins, Mr.
Hawkins, Mr. G.
Hawkins, Mr. Griffin, York-place, Clapton.
Haworth, Mr. J. Ivory-place.
Haycroft, Mr. J. S.
Haynes, Mr.
Heapley, Mr. Stock Exchange, London.
Heatley, Mr. 12, New-steine.
Heathcote, Mr. Tottenham.
Heathcote, Mrs. Tottenham.
Heaven, Mrs.
Hector, Mr. T. Westminster.
Helps, Mr. London.
Henniques, Mr. A. Q. London.
Hervey, Mrs. Edward.
Herbert, Mrs. 56, King's-road.
Hetherington, Mrs.
Hewetson, Mr. Croydon.
Heynes, Mrs.
Hibbert, Mr. Charles, Grove-house, Tottenham.
Hick, Mr. C. W. Cheapside, London.
Higgin, Mr. 18, German-place.
Higgin, Mrs. 18, German-place.

Higgs, Mr. John, Reading.
Hills, Mr. Crescent-street.
Hills, Mr. J. Ely, Isle of Ely.
Hill, Mr. 6, Bray's-buildings, Islington.
Hillersdon, Mr. Barnes, Surrey.
Hilton, Mr. Lime-street, London.
Hinde, Miss.
Hitchwell, Mr.
Hockley, Mr. 42, King's-road.
Hodgson, Mr. Dean's-yard, Westminster.
Hodgson, Mr. W.
Hodgton, Mr.
Hogard, Mrs,
Hole, Mr. Leicester.
Holdsworth, Mr. F. H. 3, Lincoln's-Inn.
Hollis, Mr. Geo.
Holland, Mr.
Holland, Mr. St. James's-street.
Holland, Mr. F.A.S. 7, Essex-street, London.
Holland, Mrs. 45, Grand-parade.
Holroyd, Mr. Barkham, Sussex.
Holt, Mr. G. P.
Homfray, Mr. Jeston.
Homewood, Mr.
Honpaye, Mr. 7, Conduit-street, Hanover-square, London.
Hope, Mr. W. Rathbone-place, London.
Hood, Mr.
Horne, Mr. 58, Regency-square.
Hornby, Mr. Steine-hotel.
Hordern, Mr. Sardon, Staffordshire.
Houghton, Miss.
Houre, Mrs.
Houssemayne Du Boulay, Mrs. Hornsey.
Howell, Mr. London.
Hubball, Mrs. Thomas, Turnham-green.
Huges, Mrs.

Hull, Mr. Uxbridge.
Hullah, Mr. A. Holborn.
Humphrey, Mr. E. Chichester.
Hurst, Mrs. 9, Broad-street.
Hurry, Mr. Edward, London.
Hutchinson, Mr. London.
Hymer, Mr. 4, Crescent.
Hindham, Mr. C. Brompton.

Irving, Major, 32, Steine.
Impey, Edward.
Impey, Mr. E. Newick:
Ind, Mr. Cambridge.
Inge, Mr. Thorpe, Staffordshire.
Innell, Mr. J. D. Long-acre, London.
Innes, Mr. John, London.
Insoll, Mr. Lewes.
Ingram, Mr.
Inwood, Mrs. Euston-square, London.
Irvine, Mr.

Jackson, Lady.
Jackson, Rev. Mr.
Jackson, Mr. R.
Jacks, Mr. Western-place.
Jacques, Mr. John, East-cliff.
James, Mr. Westminster.
James, Mr. R. Leyton, Essex.
Jameson, Miss, Haymarket, London.
Jaques, Mr. G. London.
Jaques, Mr. J. S. Homerton.
Jaques, Mr. Tottenham, Middlesex.
Jaques, Mrs. Tottenham, Middlesex.
Jarvis, Mr. R. Longacre, London.
Jarvis, Miss, Haddenham, near Thame, Oxfordshire.
Jeffrys, Miss.

Jen, Mr. Thomas, London.
Jenkins, Mr.
Jenkins, Mr. Navy-office, London.
Jennings, Mr. W. D. Great Knight Rider-street, London
Jennis, Mr. John, Maresfield.
Jervoise, Mr.
Jerlin, Mr. John Inglis.
Jerdein, Mr. M. London.
Johnson, Mr. W. 43, Aldermanbury, London
Johnstone, Mr. R. New-street-square, London.
Johnstone, Mr. Norfolk-street, London.
Jolly, Mr.
Jones, Mr. C. London.
Jones, Mr. J. Staines.
Jones, Mr. W. R.
Jones, Miss, 26, Bedford-square.
Jones, Mrs. Regency-square.
Jones, Mrs. Leytonstone, Essex.
Jones, Mrs. Milbank, Westminster.
Jones, Mr. W. Croydon.
Joy, Mr. Cheam.
Joy, Mr. Best's Boarding-house.
Jowett, Mr.
Judkins, 30, King's-road.
Jupp, Miss, Goring, Sussex.

Knightley, Lady.
Kennedy, Hon. Mrs. 27, Marine-parade.
Knox, Hon. Capt. R.N.
Kater, Capt.
Knyvett, Rev. C. W. Dean-yard, Westminster.
Kelly, Rev. A. P.
Kenny, Dr.
Kaye, Mr. Wandsworth-common, Surry.
Kelly, Mr. Cambridge.
Kelly, Mr. J. D. Cheltenham.

Kell, Mr. N. P. Battel.
Keates, Mr. J. 30, King's-road.
Kersey, Mr.
Keeling, Mr. H. 15, Marine-street.
Keen, Mr. Croydon.
Kennedy, Mr. T. from Switzerland.
Kennedy, Mr. Snaresborough, Essex.
Kemp, Mr. W.
Kemp, Mr.
Kemp, Mrs.
Kettle, Mr.
Keyser, Mr. R.A. Finsbury-square.
Killespie, Mr. Temple, London.
King, Mr. East-Blachington.
King, Mr. W.
King, Mr. Josh.
King, Mr. Stamford-hill.
Kimber, Mr. J. J.
Kirley, Mr. G. Appletree, Northamptonshire.
Kimpton, Mr. Ware.
Knight, Mr. Chelmsford.
Kneller, Mr. 69, Marine-parade.
Knatchbull, Mr. Thomas, 10, Broad-street.
Knox, J. H.
Kramer, Mr. C.

Leeds, Duchess of.
Lake, Hon. Mrs. York-hotel.
Lansdowne, Lord.
Lismore, Dean of.
Le Mesurier, Col.
Le Mesurier, Capt.
Le Mesurier, Lieut. R.N.
Le Mesurier, Miss L.
Le Blanc, Miss, E.
Lawson, Sir W.

Loundes, Dr.
Leryiantion, Captain, Coldstream Guards.
Laay, Mr. High-Wycombe, Bucks.
Lackington, Mr. 24, New-Steine.
Lacy, Mr. S. East-lane, Bermondsey.
Lacy, Mr. J. H. London.
Laire, Mr. G.
Lamport, Mr. Oxfordshire.
Lambe, Mrs. 22, Marine-parade.
Lamb, Mr. Augustus, Melbourne-lodge, Marine-parade.
Lambeth, Mr. J. Whittle, Essex.
Lancaster, Mr. S. J. Norwood.
Lane, Miss.
Lane, Mr. J. T.
Lang, Mr. 16, King's-road.
Langford, Miss.
Langford, Mr. R.
Lapidge, Mr. E.
Lapp, Mr. Cork, Ireland.
Larock, Mr. J.
Lascelles, Iremonger, Mrs. and Miss.
Latham, Mr. S. 15, Cannon-place.
Latimer, Mr. Greville-street, Brunswick-square, London.
Lavic, Mrs.
Lawrence, Mr.
Layton, Mrs.
Leake, M. H. M.P. Dorset-street, Portland-place.
Leader, Master M. 79, Wells-street, Oxford-street, London.
Leaf, M. W. Peckham-rye Green, Surry.
Lechmares, Miss.
Ledger, Mr. John.
Lee, Miss.
Lee, Mr. Weymouth-street, Portland-place.
Leete, Mr. East-cliff.
Lemmé, Mons. from Frankfort.
Letts, Mr. Thomas, Clapham, Surry.

Lierlies, Mr.
Leslie, Mr. New-steine-hotel.
Les Voeux, Mr.
Lewin, Mr. 100, King's-road.
Levesque, Mr.
Liburne, Mr. 60, Marine-parade.
Lightfoot, Mr. Old Burlington-street, London.
Light, Mr. Doctor's Commons.
Lindsay, Mr. G.
Lindsay, Mr. Queen-street, London.
Lingham, Mr. Shooter's-hill, Kent.
Lingham, Miss, M. King's-road.
Linch, Mr. D. A. 46, Steine.
Lindo, Mr.
Littledale, Mr. Best's Boarding-house.
Lloyd, Mr. J. Leatherhead, Surry.
Lloyd, Mr.
Lloyd, Mr. R. Teddington.
Lloyd, Mr. Henry, 11, Pavilion-parade.
Lloyd, Mr. J. jun. Nelson-square, London.
Lochier, Miss, 51, King's-road.
Loder, Mr.
Long, Mr. W. Steine-hotel.
Loncy, Mr.
Loudon, Mr.
Lonsdale, Mr. J. B.
Low, Mr. Surgeon, Kent-road.
Lovett, Mr. Club-house, Brighton.
Lovell, Rev. Mr.
Loveless, Mr. 18, Grenville-place.
Loughton, Mr. Fareham, Hants.
Luck, Mr. J. Battel.
Lucas, Mr. Warwick-street, London.
Lucas, Mr. Mathew P. of Lee.
Loundes, Mr. 3, Cannon-place.
Lutyens, Mr. A. L. Brixburne, Herts.

Luttaby, Mr.
Lycett, Mr. Birmingham.
Lycott, Mr. Birmingham.
Lyde, Mr.
Lysons, Rev. Mr.
Lyon, Mr. James, Brixton.
Lyon, Mr. 4, Princes-street.

Mexborough, Countess of.
Maitland, Mrs. Admiral.
Monson, Lord.
Mountcharles, Lord.
Middleton, Lord, Nottinghamshire.
Middleton, Lady, Nottinghamshire.
Malcolm, Lady.
Malcolm, Capt. R.N.
Malcolm, Sir Pulteney.
Macdonald, Hon. A.
Munro, Major-General, Grand-parade.
Macdonald, esq. M.P.
Mercer, Lieut-Col.
Macpherson, Lieutenant-Colonel, Marine-hotel.
Meyrick, Lieutenant-Colonel.
Martin, Major, Best's Boarding-house.
Moody, Major, R.E.
Macpherson, Mr. Surgeon to H.R.H. the Duke of York.
Macpherson, Capt.
Maples, Captain, R.N.
Maxwell, Rev. W. G.
Mitchell, Rev. E. D. 101, Borough.
Melville, Rev. R. Leslie.
Majendie, Rev. G. West-cliff-house.
Middleton, Rev. H.
Maltby, Dr. Buckden, Huntingdonshire.
Magnay, Alderman.
Magnay, M. W. College-hill, London.

Magnay, Mr. C. J.
Magnay, Mr. J.
Magnay, Mr. W.
Macdonald, Mr. L.
Macdonald, Mr. A.
Macdonald, Mr. John.
Macdonnell, Mr.
Mackenzie, Mr. J.
Mackinlay, Mrs. 39, West-cliff.
Mactaggalt, Mr. Upper Berkeley-street, Portland-place, London.
Macle, Mr. John.
Macculloch, Mr.
Macpherson, Mrs. 25, Marine-parade.
Mc'Gaub, Mr. C. 14, Wimpole-street.
Madocks, Mr. John, Denbigh.
Mallard, Mr. Hampstead.
Malonek, Mr. J. W. Liverpool.
Manley, Mr. James, Paternoster-row, London.
Mann, Mr. H. Prince's-street, Bank.
Manning, Mrs.
Manning, Mrs. F.
Marcuard, Mrs.
Marillier, Mr. J. W. Harrow.
Marwick, Mr. T. Firle.
Marlton, Miss.
Marlton, Mr. King's-road.
Marmaduke, Mr. Hurst.
Marryat, Mr. Joseph.
Marshall, Mr. L. London.
Marshall, Mr. John, London.
Marten, Miss.
Martin, Miss.
Martin, Miss, Helvedon, Essex.
Martin, Mr. Matthew, East-hoathly.
Marsden, Mr. Richard, London.

Maseyk, Mr.
Mason, Mr. S. Wimbledon, Surry.
Mascall, Mr. E. J. Collector of His Majesty's Customs, London.
Mather, Mr. W. Dover.
Mathews, Mr. Thames-street, London.
Matyear, Mr. G.
Maude, Mr. S. D. Brunswick-street, Islington.
Maude, Mrs.
Mawhood, Mr. 10, East-cliff.
Maxey, Mr. Northampton.
Maxse, Mr.
Maynard, Mrs.
Maynard, Miss.
Mayhew, Mr. Joshua, 7, Great Marlborough-street.
Meacham, Mr. Critchel.
Melbold, Mr.
Melbourne, Miss P.
Melville, Mr. A. 24, Upper Harley-street, London.
Melmor, Miss.
Menzies, Mr. J. Edinburgh.
Menet, Mr. J. F. Lower Rock Gardens.
Mercer, Mr.
Merricks, Mr. Chichester.
Mesman, Mr.
Meyer, Mr. F.
Meyer, Mrs. Red Lion Square, London.
Meyrick, Mr.
Middleton, Mrs. Walton-upon-Thames.
Midlane, Mr. C. W. H. J.
Miley, Mr. 60, Church-street.
Miller, Mr. Bond-street.
Milner, Mr. Old Change, London.
Mitchell, Mr. W. Upper Harley-street, London.
Mitchell, Mr. J. Wimpole-street, London.
Mitchell, Mr. Forbes.
Mitchell, Mr. Peckham-rye, Surry.

Mitchell, Mr. Edward, Croydon.
Moate, Mr. Joseph.
Mocatta, Mrs.
Mocklin, Mr.
Moffat, Mr.
Moffatt, Mrs. 41, King's-road.
Money, Mrs. cured of a swelling in the chest.
Monk, Mr. Lewis.
Monkton, Mr. 20, Regency-square.
Montdew, Mrs.
Montague, Mr. Edward.
Montgomerie, Mr. 51, Baker-street, London.
Montgomerie, Mr. Molineux.
Moore, Mrs. Calvert.
Moore, Mr. 10, Cannon-place.
Moore, Mr. G. Carey-street, Lincoln's Inn.
Moon, Mr. J. 62, Green-street, Grosvenor-square, London.
Moreton, Mr. 52, Baker-street, London.
Mordgen, Mr. Thomas.
Morgan, Mr. Octavius, 52, Regency-square.
Morgan, Mr. W. Camberwell.
Morgan, Mrs. Grand-parade.
Morrice, Mr. London.
Morrice, Mr. South-street, London.
Morris, Miss.
Morris, Mr. V. Old Ship.
Morant, Mr. J. G. Old Ship.
Morse, Mr. 14, New-steine.
Morel, Miss.
Moses, Mr. J. Wandsworth-road.
Moseley, Mr. W.
Moseley, Mr. R. London.
Mould, Mr. R. A. 70, East-street.
Mountain, Mrs. John, St. Martin's-lane.
Muggridge, Mrs.
Murray, Mr. C. K.

Murthwaite, Miss.
Mutrie, Mr. Peckham-rye, Surry.
Murphy, Mr. 7, Marine-parade.

Nagle, Sir E.
Newark, Viscount.
Nugent, Sir James.
Norton, Hon. Miss.
Newberry, Captain, 14, German-place.
Nash, Mr. John, Windsor.
Nash, Mr. Joseph, Reigate.
Naghten, Mr. Old Ship.
Nailer, Mr. Joseph, 65, Grand-parade.
Napier, Miss Emily, 70, King's-road.
Neale, Mrs.
Neate, Mr. Devonshire-place.
Neave, Miss, 23, West-cliff.
Newcastle, Mr. Stanhope-street.
Newland, Mr.
Newton, Mr. Clapham Common.
Newton, Mr. M. L. 9, Charles-street.
Netherwood, Mr. Miles, 37, Dorset-gardens.
Nicholls, Mr. J. Kensington.
Nicole, Mr. Fenchurch-street, London.
Nicholl, Mr.
Nicholl, Mrs.
Normansell, Mr.
Norris, Mr. James, London.
North, Mr. R. G.
Noy, Mr. E. H. Tower-street.

Osborne, Lady Charlotte.
Ogg, Major-General, Grove-house, Acton.
Orde, General, Marine Hotel.
O'Brien, Mrs.

Occleston, Mr. Manchester.
O'Connor, Mr. D. Hackney.
Oliver, Mr. N. 197, Holborn.
Olliver, Mrs.
Olliver, W. East Preston.
Ollive, Mr.
Ongley, Mr.
Orbell, Mr. J. Bury St. Edmunds.
Oving, Mr. G. Chichester.
Owen, Mr. J. J. Guildford.
Oxhenham, Mr.
Oxinford, Miss.

Paulet, Lady Henry.
Pindar, Lady Charlotte, Old-steine, at the Countess of Clonmell's.
Pringle, Lady, West-cliff-lodge.
Pigot, Lady, Regency-square.
Pigott, General.
Pigott, Captain, R. N.
Pigott, Admiral, Beddington, Surry.
Prudhoe, Lord.
Pelham, Lord.
Peacocke, Lieutenant-General Sir Warren.
Pallatt, Lord.
Pawlett, Major-General, 41, Steine.
Pierpoint, Colonel, Ryhall, Rutland.
Phillott, Major.
Pym, Sir Henry.
Paul, Sir John, Bart.
Pryce, Captain, Bengal Artillery.
Phillimon, Captain.
Poulett, Captain.
Price, Captain, R. N.
Paterson, Capt.
Paget, Captain, Chichester.

Pain, Mr. North Brixton.
Palmer, Mr. Thomas, 12, Holborn-court, London.
Palmer, Mr. P.
Panton, Mr. Andrew, Cheapside, London.
Parey, Mr. Welbeck-street, London.
Parker, Mr.
Parker, Mrs.
Parkinson, Mr.
Parkinson, Mr. J. T.
Parkinson, Miss.
Parkinson, Mrs. 22, Lower-rock-gardens.
Paronall, Mrs. German-place.
Parlett, Mrs.
Parlett, Mr. James.
Parlet, Mr. W. Madehurst.
Pasker, Mr.
Patching, Miss E.
Paterson, Mr. Temple, London.
Patre, Mr. Wimpole-street, London.
Pattulto, Mr. W.
Paul, Mr. R. C. Norfolk-house.
Paul, Mr. West-cliff House.
Paxton, A. Kensington.
Paynder, Mr. J. London.
Payne, Mr.
Paynter, Mr.
Payne, Mr. B. M. Camelford-street.
Peake, Mrs.
Peare, Mrs.
Peavee, Mrs.
Peirse, Mr. Norfolk-hotel.
Perkins, Mr. Bath.
Perkins, Mr. Henry, Springfield, Surry.
Perry, Mrs.
Perry, Mr.
Perry, Mr. G.

Peters, Mr. Borough.
Peters, Mr. jun. Borough:
Petre, Mr. Welbeck-street, London.
Petty, Mr. London.
Phelan, Mr. London.
Phelan, Mr. John, London.
Phillips, Mr. Tottenham.
Philipott, Mr. Kensington-gardens.
Phipps, Mr. Dorking.
Phipps, Mr. J.
Pike, Charles, Dalston.
Pike, Mr. B. W. London.
Pine, Mr. Islington.
Piray, Miss.
Pitter, Mr. J. R. Bedford-street, Covent-garden.
Pittcock, Mr. R. Tunbridge-wells.
Pitman, Mr. Marine-hotel.
Plouden, Mr. R. C. York-hotel.
Plumer, Mrs.
Pockington, Mr. Cumberland.
Pollard, Mr. James.
Pomfrett, Mr. J. D.
Poingdestre, Mr. Best's Boarding-house.
Poole, Mr. Homerton, Middlesex.
Pott, Mr. A.
Pownell, Mr. John, jun.
Powle, Mr. S. C.
Powell, Mr. Dane Hill.
Power, Mr. P.
Pousett, Mr. H. 226, Upper Thames Street, London.
Prater, Mr. W. Arlington-street, St. James's,
Prater, Mr. A.
Pratt, E.
Price, Mr. London.
Price, Mr. R.
Pringle, Mrs. and Miss, 2, German-place.

Prince, Mr. J. Haymarket.
Priest, Mr. Bow-street, St. George's-street, Bryanstone-square, London.
Prier, Mr. J. W. Newington.
Prina, Mr. John, 19, Marine-parade.
Proctor, Mr. G. Mardock, Herts.
Proixdo, Mr.
Prosser, Mrs. Southwark.
Pryor, Mr. N. London.
Pugh, Mr. Bernard-street, Russell-street, London
Purcell, Mr. Shoreham.
Pyne, Mr. Henry, Ludgate-street, London.

Quin, Lord George.

Reay, Lord.
Reardon, Honourable, Mrs.
Radcliffe, Lieutenant-Colonel.
Robbins, Lieutenant-Colonel, Steine-hotel.
Rosenberg, Mr. Messenger to the King.
Russell, Rev. Dr.
Ridge, Captain
Rodd, Captain
Roberts, Captain
Roddy, Captain, 89th Regiment.
Rawlins, Rev. Christopher.
Raikes, Mr. J.
Raikes, Mrs. Richard Mee.
Ralli, Mr. 18, Camomile-street.
Rathbone, Miss
Rawlins, Mr. S. W. Liverpool-street.
Ravenscroft, Mrs.
Raymond, Mr. London.
Rayward, Mr. Lewes, Sussex.
Real, Mr. A. Tunbridge Wells.
Redhouse, Mr. Robert.

Reeves, Mr. I. London
Rehn, Mr.
Reid, Mr. London
Reid, Mr. E. Southampton
Reid, Mr. G. A. 2d Life Guards
Reiwall, Mr. F. 56, King's-road
Renalds, Miss
Rennie, Mr.
Rendall, Mr. H. E.
Re w, Mr. I. London
Reynolds, Mr. M.D.
Rhoades, Mr. W. C. Chichester
Rhoades, Mr. T. Chichester
Rhoades, Mr. Edward, Chichester
Rhodes, Miss, 57, Marine-parade
Richards, Mr. F. St. Martin's-lane, London
Richardson, Mrs.
Riette, Mr. A. London
Rigley, Mr. Nottingham
Rigby, Mr. Hoxton
Riddle, Mrs.
Rider, Miss
Robbins, Mr. W.
Robins, Mr. Joseph
Robley, Mr. John-street
Robinson, Mr. S. Saffron Walden, Essex
Robinson, Mr. R. London
Roch, Mr. R.
Roche, Mr. R. Green-coat-row, Westminster
Rogers, Mr. John
Roles, Mr. Grey-coat-street, Westminster
Ronalds, Mr.
Roper, Mr. A.
Rothery, Mr. W. P.
Rose, Mr. John
Rotton, Mrs. Newington-green

Rouse, Mrs.
Rousseau, Mr. P. C. S.
Rowles, Mr. Henry
Rowe, Mr. I. Petworth
Rowell, Miss
Rowen, Mrs. Pentonville
Russell, Miss
Rutter, Mr. T. Mordon, Surry
Rutter, Mr. Mitcham, Surry

Stewart, Lady
Strachan, Lady
Stuart, Lady
Stuart, Lady Elizabeth
Stepney, Lady, 1, Prince's-street
Sheffield, Dowager Lady, Portman-street, London
Shepperd, Lady Mary, 26, Marine-parade
Somerset, Lady Louisa
Seymour, Lady Charlotte, 62, King's-road
Sotheron, Admiral
St. John, Hon. General
Smith, General
Smith, Mrs. Colonel, 31, Grand-parade
Serle, Colonel
Stumpt, Major
Sandham, Major
Skelton, Major
Shelley, Sir John
Stopford, Sir Robert
Stewart, Mr. M.P.
Saunders, Captain
Sykes, Captain T.
Shepheard, Capt.
Stoddart, Dr.
Styles, Dr.
Shepherd, Rev. H.

Smirgrove, Rev. J. Welbeck-street, London.
Smith, Lieut. R. N. Guildford.
Snow, Rev. Mr.
Stoughton, Rev. Mr.
Sturges, Rev. Mr.
Scott, Rev. Mr. Malton-street.
Scobell, Rev. Mr. S.
Saumarez, Rev. J.
Sadler, Mr. R.
Sadle, Mr.
Sage, Mr. G.
Saloway, Mr. London.
Samuel, Mr. Simon, 16, Bedford-square.
Sandley, Mr.
Sandys, Mr. Thomas, Vauxhall.
Sandon, Mr. S.
Sanctuary, Mrs. 27, New -steine.
Sarel, Mr. Berkeley-square.
Saunt, Mr. 6, Ship-street.
Saunders, Miss, 4, New-steine.
Sanderson, Mr. Norbury-house, near Croydon.
Saurin, Miss Emily, 7, Pavilion-parade.
Savage, Mr. B. 18, Bedford-street.
Savage, Mr. 12, East-cliff.
Saville, Mr. Hartley.
Sawyer, Mr. J. Horsham.
Sayer, Mr. 70, Marine-parade.
Scade, Mrs.
Scaley, Mr. Trinity-square, London.
Scaith, Mr. Star and Garter Hotel.
Scholey, Mr. G. Clapham Common, Surry.
Scott, Mr. Thomas, Stonehurst.
Schneider, Miss.
Scott, Mr. W. Bartholomew-lane.
Searle, Mr. Saffron Walden.
Searle, Mr. J.

Seddon, Mrs. G.
Sedgwick, Miss.
Serony, Mrs.
Sewell, Mr. J.
Severrs, Mr. Thomas, 18, Grand-parade.
Seymour, Miss.
Sharp, Mr. High-street, Mary-le-bone, London.
Sharp, Mr. H. Kew.
Sharp, Mr. Samuel, 5, Essex-court, Temple.
Sharp, Mr. G. A. Tavistock-street.
Sharpe, Mr. F. Temple, London.
Shalto, Mrs. Duncombe, West Lodge.
Shaplin, Mr. 3, New-steine.
Shafto Gornault, Mr. Robert.
Shee, Mr.
Sheppard, Mr. Hampstead.
Sheppard, Mr. W. 15, East-cliff.
Sherborne, Mr. Bedford-square, Middlesex.
Sherwood, Mr. W.
Sherwood, Mr. Thomas.
Shirley, Mrs. Evelyn.
Shipley, Mr.
Shucht, Mr. G. London.
Shulto, Mr. W. Southbank, St. Johns.
Simpson, Miss.
Simpson, Mr. D. London.
Simpson, Mr. W.
Sims, Mr. W. N.
Sinales, Mr.
Skelton, Mr. Hampstead.
Skene, Lieut.
Skipper, Mr. C. London.
Skinner, Mr. 5, West-cliff.
Slack, Mr. W. Cheapside, London.
Slack, Mr. W. Jun. ditto, ditto.
Slater, Mr. F. London.

Slater, Mr. J. Haselback, Northamptonshire.
Slaney, Mr. London.
Slade, Mr. W.
Smart, Mr.
Smallpiece, Mr. Job, near Guildford.
Smelt, Mr. C. Wings, Bucks.
Smirke, Mr. R.
Smith, Mr. R.A. Woolwich.
Smith, Mr. Purley.
Smith, Mrs.
Smith, Mr. J.
Smith, Mr. T. Brentford.
Smith, Mr. C. G.
Smith, Mr. W. London.
Smith, Mr. W. Southville, Wandsworth Road.
Smith, Mr. S. sen. Clay-street Cottage, Walthamstow, Essex.
Smithson, Mr.
Smythe, Mr. W.
Smythe, Miss.
Smythe, Mr. C.
Smilly, Mr. 8, Marine-parade.
Snellgrove, Mr. London.
Snowdon, Mr. P.
Southerby, Mrs. and Miss
Southall, Mr.
Spalding, W. D. Camberwell.
Spalding, Mr. C. W. Camberwell.
Sparkes, Mr. Stoke, near Guilford.
Spragg, Mr. George, 20, King's-road.
Spence, Mrs. Malling-house, near Lewes.
Spring, Mr. Southampton, Hants.
Spiller, Mr. R.
Spitty, Mr. T.
Spinner, Mr. T. Old-ship.
Spurr, Mrs.
Spurr, Mr. 1, Grafton-place.

Stables, Miss, 28, Steine.
Stables, Miss L.
Stanford, Mr. Preston.
Stanes, Mr. James, 12, East-cliff.
Stapleton, Mr. and Mrs.
Starling, G. Brewer-street, London.
Stansfield, Mr. T. 42, Steine.
Steinbach, Mr. George.
Stephens, Mr. A.
Stephens, Mr. Uxbridge.
Stephens, Mr. 4, East-cliff.
Stephenson, Mr. and Mrs.
Stephenson, Mr. C. D. 1, Moore-place, Lambeth, Surry.
Stevens, Mr. H. J.
Stevenson, Mr. G. Clapham.
Steel, Mr. Thomas, Old-ship.
Stewart, Mr. James, London.
Stewart, Mr. Jermyn-street, London.
Stewart, Miss.
Stokes, Mr.
Stooks, Mr. T.
Stone, Mr. Bennet's-place, Gracechurch-street, London.
Stovell, Mrs. G. 17, King's-road.
Street, Mr. Pavilion-parade.
Sterling, Mrs. Battersea.
Sterling, Mr. T. H. 60, Grand-parade.
Strongitham, Mr. J. 38, Regency-square.
Strettell, Mr. W. T. 12, Devonshire-place.
Sturgis, Mrs. and Miss, 5, King's-road.
Stuart, Miss Louisa, York-hotel.
Stuart, Mr. John, Windsor.
St. Leger, Miss
Sullivan, Mr. W.
Sumner, Mrs. Holme.
Surman, Miss.
Sutherland, Mr. Gloucester-place, London.

Swain, Mr. Hertford.
Swimer, Mr. W. John-street, Berkeley-square, London.
Symons, Mr.

Tierney, Lady, Pavilion-parade
Titchfield, Marquis
Tyrconnel, Earl of
Travers, Major-General
Trench, Colonel
Thornton, Colonel
Tierney, Rev. M.A. Arundel
Tredcroft, Rev. E. Pulborough
Talbot, Hon. T. C. 9, New-steine
Taite, Mr: J. Oxford-street, London
Taite, Mrs. 3, King's-road
Tanner, Mr. James
Tatham, Mrs. J.
Taylor, Mr. J. H. 4, Great Queen's-street, Westminster
Taylor, Mr. Simon.
Taylor, Mr. R. Valparaiso
Tayton, Mr.
Tenbroche, Mr.
Tendal, Mr.
Tergus, Mr. W. London
Thetford, Mr.
Theobald, Mr. Upper Brook-street, Grosvenor-square, London
Thomson, Mr. F. C.
Thomson, Mr. J.
Thomson, Mr. Robert, East-grinstead
Thomson, Mr. Samuel, Plaistow, Essex
Thomson, Mr. W. Bedford-place
Thomson, Mr. R. 42, Steine
Thornton, Mrs. 61, King's-road
Thwynce, Mrs.
Tibbits, Mr. Barton, Sea-grove, near Kettering
Tidd, Mr. John, Wigmore-street, London

Tidswell, Mr. R.
Tillstone, Mr. J. Moulscombe-place, Sussex
Tindall, Miss
Todd, Mr. W.
Toemas, Mr. R. 62, Grand-parade
Toghill, Mr. Chichester
Tood, Mr. T. London
Toussaint, Mr. and Mrs. 47, King's-road
Trail, Mr. H. York-hotel
Trevett, Mr. R. London
Treedell, Mr. L. W. Stepney
Trickey, Mr. S. 6, Richmond-place
Trucy, Mrs. and Miss
Trueman, Mr. T. London
Tuck, Mrs.
Tulk, Mr.
Tunnard, Mr. W.
Tuplin, Mr. W.
Turnbull, Mr.
Turner, Mr. Michael, 40, Bloomsbury-place
Turner, Mr. Skinner, 40, Bloomsbury-place
Tusm, W. Limehouse
Twisleton, Miss

Ume, Sir A.
Unwin, Mr.
Upton, Major-General
Upton, Mr. E. Croydon
Urquhart, Mrs. 13, Bedford-square
Usborne, Mrs. 41, Marine-parade

Vice-Chancellor the, York-hotel
Vansitzozely Detvitrych, from Antwerp
Vyner, Capt.
Vanoven, Mr. A. London
Vaughan, Mr. G. 82, Grand-parade

Vaughan, Mrs. 5, German-place
Valentine, Mr.
Vardon, Mr. W. Gracechurch-street
Vassall, Mr. Lymington
Vernon, Mr. C.
Villiers, Mr.
Vincent, Mrs.
Vyner, Miss and Miss C.

Wellington, His Grace the Duke of
Wortley, Lady Caroline
Whitshed, Lady
Weld, Hon. Mrs. H. Chidcock-house, Dorset
Wells, Vice-Admiral
Wellesley, Sir Henry
Wilder, Sir F.
Watson, Sir W: H. 6, East-cliff
Way, Col. Sir Gregory
Wombwell, Sir George
Wynn, Sir William
Wyndham, Colonel
Woodford, Colonel, 70, King's-road
Whatley, Colonel
West, Lieutenant-Colonel
Wallis, Lieutenant-Colonel, B. York Hotel
Willard, Major
Watson, Major D.
Walwyn, Major
Woodley, Captain, R.N.
Worth, Captain John, R.N. 20, Regent-place.
Worth, Captain, R.N. Oakley, Suffolk
Williams, Captain, R.N.
Webb, Captain, Steine Hotel
Watkinson, Rev. R. Charter-house.
Wilson, Rev. G. Norfolk
West, Rev. Mr. 16, New-steine

Wynter, Dr.
Wain, Mr. J. 67, St. James's-street, London
Wake, Mr. Millbank, Westminster
Wake, Miss, 1, Pavilion-parade
Walker, Mr. and Mrs. C. Kensington Grove
Walker, Miss M. Gestingthorpe
Wallace, Mr. J. L.
Wallace, Mr. P. Petersham, Surry
Wallace, Mr. George, Paradise-house, Stoke Newington
Wallace, Mr. and Mrs.
Wallaston, Mr. London
Wall, Mr. G. London
Wall, Mrs. Kenilworth
Waller, Mr. John, Long Acre
Wallington, Mr. G.
Wallis, Mr. J. Portslade
Walters, Mr. Marine Hotel
Walton, Mr. W.
Walsham, Mr. Charles, Ashted Lodge, Surry
Walsham, Mr. C.
Ward, Miss, 6, Devonshire-place
Wardle, Mr. T.
Wares, Mr. S. Hampstead
Waring, Mrs.
Warman, Miss, West-cliff-house
Warnum, Miss, 9, German-place
Warwick, Mr. Charles, London
Warwick, Miss M. 17, Devonshire-place
Watson, Mr. Hampstead
Watson, Mr. W. G.
Watson, Mr. and Mrs.
Waterhouse, Mr. B. G. London
Watts, Mr. Thomas, Bunhill-row, London
Wattleworth, Mr.
Way, Miss Catherine
Webb, Mr. Plaskett, Essex

Webb, Mr. T. Waterloo-road
Webb, Mr. T. G. Ware, Herts.
Weldon, Mr. Charles
Weldon, Mr. J.
Welsh, Mr. J. M. Pine's Hill, Essex
Weller, Mr. New Ship Inn, Brighton.
West, Mr. J.
West, Mr.
Westbrook, Mr. J.
Westmacott, Mr. H. 34, Cadogan-place
Weymark, Mr. M.
Weymark, Mr.
Whalby, Mrs.
Wheeler, Miss
Whitbread, Mr. Edmonton
White, P. Berner's-street, London
White, Mr. J. L.
White, Mr. J. Wardour-street, Soho, London
White, Mr.
White, Mrs.
White, Mr. London
White, Mr. T.
Whitehead, Mr. E. H.
Whitehead, Mr.
Whiting, Mr. C.
Whitten, Mr. R. London
Wightman, Mr.
Wigron, Mr. C.
Wildey, Mr. Hants
Wilkes, Mr. John, Lofts Hall, Essex
Wilkes, Mrs.
Wilkinson, Mr. C. W. Ship Hotel
Wilkinson, Mr. Thomas, 2, Devonshire-place, Edgeware-road, London
Willard, Miss, 46, Ship-street
Willes, Mr. Grand-parade

Williams, Miss, Bellevue-house, Brighton
Williams, Mr. Finsbury-place, London
Williams, Mr. H. W.
Williams, Mrs. L. W.
Williams, Miss E. 22, Marine-parade
Williams, Mr. E. Enfield
Wilmot, Mr. London
Wilshire, Mr. Hitchin, Herts
Wilson, Miss
Wilson, Mr. Nottingham
Wilson, Mr. M.
Winborn, Mr. R. London
Windsor, Mr. H.
Winter, Miss, 52, Old-steine
Wirmall, Mr. Old Ship Hotel
Withers, Mr. R. 62, Ship-street
Wood, Mr. Thomas, Walworth
Wood, Mrs.
Wood, Mr. 98, King's-road
Wooden, Miss
Woodley, Mr. W. London
Woodman, Mr. 168, Piccadilly
Woodthorpe, Mr. H. J. Guildhall, London
Woodward, Mr.
Woodward, Mr. J.
Woodward, Mr. G.
Woodward, Mrs.
Woodford, Mr. Richard-street, Islington
Woolaston, Mr. G. H. Clapham Common
Woolfe, Mr. J. R. Finsbury-place
Worstencroft, Mr. J. Bread-street, London
Wortley, Mr. R. L. Nottingham
Wright, Mr. J.
Wright, Mr. B. 8, Grafton-street
Wright, Mr. E.
Wriglett, Mr. 10, Crescent

Wyam, Mr. W.
Wyatt, Mr.
Wyatt, Mrs.
Wyatt, Mrs. Thelvedon, Essex
Wyndham, Mr. C.
Wynne, Mr. G.

Young, Lady
Young, Sir William
Yates, Mr.
Yates, Miss
Yates, Miss, 2, East-cliff
Yerraway, Mrs.
Youde, Mr.
Young, Mr. J. Brookhill
Young, Mr. T. W. Marine Hotel.

INDEX.

CHAP. I.

CHAP. II.

CHAP. III.

CHAP IV.

CHAP. V.

CHAP. VI.

CHAP. VII.

ADDITIONAL TESTIMONIALS SINCE THE FIRST EDITION.

CHAP. VII.

Creasy and Baker, Printers, Gazette-office, Brighton.